HARPERESSENTIALS

What to do when the unforeseen happens

Emergency situations require immediate action, and the inexperienced first aider can easily be at a loss to know what to do. This book has been designed to help the first aider cope with such situations. Major injuries are clearly distinguished from minor ones; guides to action are distinguished from explanatory information; and "dos" and "don'ts" are clearly marked, so that even the lay person can, at a glance, know what to look for and ensure the best preliminary treatment is given to the victim.

From removing splinters to coping with heart attacks, from treating headaches to dealing with victims with suspected spinal fractures, *First Aid* will be an invaluable companion in the home, office, or when traveling.

Other HarperEssentials

STRESS SURVIVAL GUIDE
UNDERSTANDING DREAMS
WINE GUIDE

HARPERESSENTIALS

First Aid

Dr. R. M. Youngson
with The Diagram Group

HarperTorch
An Imprint of HarperCollins*Publishers*

FIRST AID is intended to give general guidance on what to do in an emergency where no physician is available. If at all possible, readers should consult a physician before attempting any treatment. If that is not possible, readers should seek medical advice as soon as possible after emergency treatment. The authors, publisher, and book producer disclaim any liability arising directly or indirectly from the use of this book.

This book was originally published in 1993 by HarperCollins UK.

❦

HARPERTORCH
An Imprint of HarperCollins*Publishers*
10 East 53rd Street
New York, New York 10022-5299

First HarperTorch paperback printing: August 2003

HarperCollins ®, HarperTorch™, and ❦ ™ are trademarks of Harper-Collins Publishers Inc.

Printed in the United States of America

Visit HarperTorch on the World Wide Web at www.harpercollins.com

10 9 8 7 6 5 4 3 2 1

Introduction

There are many cases where a knowledge of first aid can be useful, and some where it is essential. From minor injuries to major emergencies, a working familiarity with first aid practice can limit injuries sustained by a victim and, in some cases, can actually save a life.

HarperEssentials First Aid is clear, informative and user-friendly. It covers a wide variety of injuries and conditions, and enables even the most inexperienced person to provide victims with immediate preliminary aid.

Emergency situations require immediate action and the inexperienced first aider can easily find him- or herself at a loss to know what to do. This book has been designed to help the first aider cope with such situations. Major injuries are clearly distinguished from minor ones; guides to action are distinguished from explanatory information; and "dos" and "don'ts" are clearly marked, so that even the lay person can, at a glance, know what to look for and ensure that the best possible preliminary treatment is given to the victim.

From removing splinters to coping with heart attacks, from treating headaches to dealing with victims with suspected spinal fractures, *HarperEssentials First Aid* will be an invaluable companion in the home, office or when traveling. However, a full First Aid Training Course is recommended for everyone and this guide purely assists in situations when no other help is available.

Contents

How to Use This Book   xiii

Procedures of First Aid   xv

1 The Signs of Life and Emergency Techniques   1

  THE SIGNS OF LIFE   1

    A Clear Airway   1

    The Circulation   4

  EMERGENCY TECHNIQUES   6

    Artificial Resuscitation   6

    External Chest Compression   9

    Resuscitation by Two People   13

    The Recovery Position   15

    Severe Bleeding and Pressure Points   19

2 Emergency Management of Serious Injuries   22

  PRINCIPLES AND RESPONSIBILITIES   22

    The Job of the First Aider   22

    Immediate Action in an Emergency   23

Specific Injuries and Conditions 25

What the Emergency Services Need to Know 27

THE HIV RISK 27

MOVING AND LIFTING VICTIMS 30

When to Move an Injured Person 30

General Rules for Lifting 32

Which Method to Use 33

One First Aider 34

Two First Aiders 40

More Than Two First Aiders 47

REMOVING CLOTHING AND HELMETS 50

Removing Clothing 50

Removing Socks 54

Removing Helmets 54

Removing a Protective Helmet 55

Removing a Full-face Crash Helmet 56

3 Major Injuries and Dangerous Conditions 58

BLEEDING 58

Wounds and External Bleeding 58

Internal Bleeding 65

BREATHING DIFFICULTIES 65

Asphyxia 66

Choking 66

Drowning 74

Fumes and Gases 76

Strangulation 78

BURNS   80
    Causes   80
    Burn Depth   80
    Burn Area   82
    Clothing on Fire   83
    High-Temperature Burns and Scalds   86
    Chemical Burns   89
    Chemical Burns of the Eye   90
    Electrical Burns   91
CIRCULATORY PROBLEMS   93
    The Circulatory System and its Function   93
    Angina   96
    Cardiac Arrest   98
    Heart Attack   100
    Shock   104
CRUSH INJURIES   108
    The Importance of Time   109
DISLOCATIONS   111
    Dislocated Shoulder   112
EXTREMES OF BODY TEMPERATURE   114
    Heatstroke   114
    Hypothermia   116
    Frostbite   118
    Heat Exhaustion   119
FRACTURES   120
    Causes and Sites of Fracture   120

Symptoms and Signs of Fracture   121

Immobilization and Management of Fractures   123

Open Fractures   124

Neck Fractures   127

Spine Fractures   130

MUSCLE INJURIES   133

General Muscle Injuries   133

4 Minor Injuries and Conditions   135

ACHES AND PAINS   135

Backache   135

Headache   136

Earache   138

Menstrual Pain   139

Sinus Pain   140

Toothache   141

BITES AND STINGS   142

Dog, Cat and Human Bites   142

Snakebites   143

Insect Bites   145

Stings   146

BLACK EYE   148

BLEEDING   149

Minor Wounds, Cuts and Grazes   150

Nosebleeds   152

Gum and Tooth Socket Bleeding   154

BURNS   156

Minor Burns and Scalds 156

Sunburn 157

FAINTING 158

FEVERS 159

FOREIGN BODIES 161

Foreign Bodies in the Ear 161

Foreign Bodies in the Eye 162

Foreign Bodies in the Nose 164

Splinters 165

NAUSEA AND VOMITING 166

Travel sickness 167

5 Dressings, Bandages and Slings **169**

DRESSINGS 169

Bandages (Adhesive Dressings) 171

Field (Sterile) Dressings 173

Gauze Dressings 175

Improvised Dressings 177

BANDAGES 177

Roller Bandages 179

Applying Roller Bandages 180

Triangular Bandages 188

Applying Triangular Bandages 189

SLINGS 193

Arm Sling 193

Elevation Sling 195

Reef Knots 197

6 Useful Aids   198

    First Aid Kit   198

    Medicines in the Home   199

    Drugs Glossary   201

How to Use This Book

For clear, safe and speedy reference, the various text components of *HarperEssentials First Aid* have been differentiated by the use of color, and important points have been highlighted using symbols.

The text shown in colored panels gives step-by-step instructions of what to do when a particular injury or condition is encountered. So that these procedures may be found quickly and easily, an alphabetical list of them has been included on pp. xv–xix.

The text not in colored panels offers basic explanatory information about the injuries and conditions, including causes, diagnostic features, and on how certain parts of the body function.

Three symbols are used throughout *Harper-Essentials First Aid* to draw attention to important points:

❖ caution: action may harm the victim, the first aider or aggravate the injury;

◆ alternative or further procedures and/or tools to be used, if the preceding method has failed, if there are complications or if a particular tool is unavailable;

◗ read on: more important text follows.

Procedures of First Aid

A

adhesive dressings,
  applying 171–172
airway
  clearing an obstruction
  from 4
  opening 3
angina attack, manage-
  ment of 96–98
arm sling, applying
  193–194
artificial resuscitation,
  giving 7–8 see also resuscitation by two people

B

backache, relieving 136
bandages, application of
  adhesive dressings,
  171–172 see also
  roller bandages;
  triangular bandages

bites
  insect 145–146
  management of 143
  snake 143–145
  see also stings
black eye, treating
  148–149
bleeding
  controlling external
  62–64, 151
  management of
  internal 65
  stopping severe
  external 20–21
blisters, dressing broken
  88
breathing, checking for 2
burns and scalds, treating
  86–87, 156–157
  see also clothing on fire;
  chemical burns; chemical
  burns of the eye

C

carbon monoxide poisoning, treating 76–77

cardiac arrest, management of 99–100

cervical collar, making and applying 128–129

chemical burn, treating 89

chemical burns of the eye, treating 90–91

chest compression
see external chest compression

choking, methods of management 68–73
abdominal thrust 70
for babies and infants 70, 73
bending and slapping 68–70
for conscious adult 68, 71
for conscious child 69, 72

coughing 68
for unconscious adult 69, 72
for unconscious child 69, 73

clothing on fire, management of 83
rapid cooling of victim 84–85
see also burns and scalds

clothing, removing 50–4

coats, jackets, shirts, vests 51
shoes or boots 53
socks 54
trousers 52

crush injuries, management of 108–111

cuts and grazes 150–152

D

dislocated shoulder, management of 113

dressings, applying field 174–175
bandages (adhesive) 171–172
gauze 176

drowning person, resuscitating a 74–75

E

ear, removing foreign bodies from 161–162

earache, relieving 139

electrical burns, treating 91–93

elevation sling, applying 195–196

emergency situations priorities 23–25

external chest compression, performing 9–12
see also resuscitation by two people

eye
  removing foreign bodies
    from 162–164
  treating chemical burns
    of 90–91

F

fainting, management of
  159
fevers, treating 160
field dressing, applying
  174–175
figure-eight bandage,
  applying 190
first aid kit, contents of
  198–199
foreign bodies in wounds
  64
foreign bodies, removing
  from the ear 161–162
  from the eye 162–164
  from the nose 164
fractures,
  management of
    123–124
  neck 127–129
  open 124–127
  spine 130–131
frostbite,
  management of 118

G

gauze dressing,
  applying 176

gum bleeding 154–156

H

headaches, relieving 137
heart attack,
  management of 102–103
heat exhaustion,
  treating 119–120
heatstroke,
  management of 115
helmets, removing 54–57
  protective helmet 55
  full-face crash helmet 56
HIV infection, avoiding
  during resuscitation 29
hypothermia 116–118

I

insect bites, treating
  145–146
internal bleeding, treating 65

L

see also thigh-bone
  fractures
lifting a victim see moving
  a victim

M

medicine cabinet,
  contents 200
menstrual pain, relieving
  139–140
minor wounds, treating 151

moving a victim with a
spine fracture/injury
48–49
on to a stretcher 46
moving a victim
methods of 34–49
cradle 37
dragging 34–35
fireman's lift 38–39
four-handed seat 40
human crutch 36
kitchen chair 42–43
piggyback 37
two-handed seat 41
see also stretchers
muscle injuries,
management of 133–134

N

nausea and vomiting,
relieving 166–167
neck fractures,
immobilizing 128
nose, removing foreign
bodies from 164
nosebleed, stopping 153

O

open fractures,
management of 124–127

P

pressure points, using to
stop bleeding 19–21

pulse, checking the 5

R

recovery position
spinal 131–132
standard 15–18
reef knots, tying 197
resuscitation by two
people 13–14
see also artificial
resuscitation; external
chest compression
roller bandages
applying to the foot and
ankle 183–184
applying around foreign
bodies 187
applying to the hand
184–185
applying to the knee or
elbow 182–183
simple spiral technique
180–181
applying to a sprained
wrist 186

S

shock,
management of 104–108
sinus pain,
methods of relieving 141
sling, applying
arm 193–194
elevation 195–196

smoke inhalation,
    treating 77–78
snakebites, management
    of 144–145
spinal recovery position
    131–132
spine fractures
    immobilizing 130–131
    moving a person with
    48–49
splinter, removing 165–166
sprained wrist, bandaging
    186
sterile unmedicated
    dressings see field
    dressing
stings, treating 146–147
strangulation, treating
    78–79
stretchers
    making improvised
    44–45
    moving a victim onto
    46
sunburn, relieving 157–158

T

toothache, methods of
    relieving 142

tooth socket bleeding,
    stopping 155–156
travel sickness, relieving
    167–168
triangular bandages
    applying figure-eight
    bandage 190
    applying to the
    foot/hand 192–193
    applying to the scalp 191
    broad bandages 189
    narrow bandages
    189–190
turning a victim
    see moving a victim

V

victim, moving with a
    spine fracture/injury
    48–49
vomiting, relieving 167

W

wounds
    foreign bodies in 64
    preventing infection of
    151–152
    see also minor wounds
wrist, sprained 186

1

The Signs of Life and Emergency Techniques

The Signs of Life

The signs of life are breathing and the pulse. In emergency situations, the following concerns take priority: 1 that the victim's airway is clear and that they are able to breathe; and 2 that the blood is circulating properly.

A CLEAR AIRWAY

THE IMPORTANCE OF AIR SUPPLY

The most urgent and immediate responsibility for any person giving first aid is to ensure that the injured person can either breathe freely or is provided artificially with an adequate supply of air. Nothing else is as important as this. Above all, the brain needs oxygen. At normal temperatures, serious brain damage or even death will occur in a matter of minutes if a person ceases to have an adequate intake of air. This may happen because the person has stopped breathing or because the passage along which the air enters the lungs (the airway) has become obstructed.

The first requirement is to check for breathing.

CHECKING FOR BREATHING

Use more than one sense: **1** look for movements of the chest or abdomen—confirm that these are smooth and regular; **2** listen close to the mouth or nose for sounds of breathing; **3** you should be able to feel the victim's breath on your face.

If the casualty is breathing freely you can safely turn your attention to checking for injuries. If the casualty is unconscious and the injuries permit, use the recovery position (see pp. 15–18) to ensure that safe breathing continues.

IF THERE IS NO BREATHING

This means that respiration has ceased and you must supply the air. If the chest and abdomen are moving, but there is no movement of air in and out of the mouth or nose, the airway is obstructed and you must clear it. Action is urgently needed to restore the air supply. Shout for help and ensure an ambulance has been called.

OPENING THE AIRWAY

1 The airway may be blocked by the position of the head (**a**). **2** To remedy this, press down on the forehead with one hand and with the

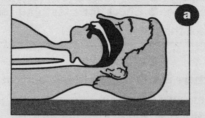

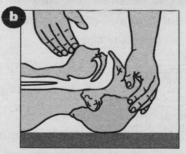

other lift the chin with two fingertips (**b**). This action stops the tongue from blocking the top of the airway.

◆ **If there is still no breathing,** there may be an obstruction in the airway.

CLEARING AN OBSTRUCTION
FROM THE AIRWAY

1 Turn the head to one side, keeping the chin forward and the top of the head back. **2** Sweep around the inside of the mouth above the tongue with two hooked fingers and remove any foreign material. Do this quickly. Do not waste time. **3** Check for breathing (see p. 2). **4** Check the pulse (opposite).

◆ **If there is still no breathing,** start artificial ventilation at once (see pp. 6–9).

◆ **If there is no breathing** *and* **no pulse,** start artificial ventilation and external chest compression (see pp. 9–12) immediately.

THE CIRCULATION

The pulse indicates the state of the circulation. It is the repeated, brief pressure wave that passes along the arteries each time the lower chambers of the heart tighten (contract) and squeeze out blood. The rate and quality of the pulse may vary considerably, from slow, full and thrusting to rapid, weak and fluttering. A rapid, weak pulse, characteristic of shock (see pp. 104–108), may be difficult to feel, especially in a panic situation where the first aider's own heart may be beating rapidly and his or her pulse may be much stronger than that of the victim.

For this reason, feeling the pulse at the usual site, on the thumb side of the wrist, 1.5 cm above the wrist crease and 1.5 cm in from the edge (a), may not be reliable. So you should always feel for the carotid pulse in the neck. The carotids are large arteries that run up on either side of the back of the Adam's apple (larynx) (b).

CHECKING THE PULSE

1 Breathe deeply to calm yourself, if necessary. **2** Use only the tips of two fingers. Place them on the side of the Adam's apple without pressing on it. **3** Slide your fingertips firmly backwards along the side of the Adam's apple so that they pass into the vertical groove between it and the muscle to the side of it (**c**). **4** If you do not immediately feel the pulse, move the ▶

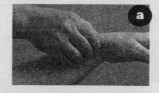

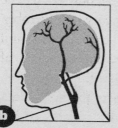

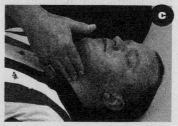

fingertips a little nearer to and further from the
Adam's apple until the pulse is felt.

Emergency Techniques

ARTIFICIAL RESUSCITATION

The object of this is to provide the victim immediately with an air supply. The air you breathe out still
has adequate amounts of oxygen for someone else to
use. Many lives have been saved with "second-hand" oxygen. There must be no delay in starting
artificial resuscitation and you must be sure that the
air is getting to the right place—deep into the lungs
of the victim.

It is essential that you succeed in inflating the
lungs. If you do not see the chest rising when you
blow and falling when you stop, you are not succeeding; you may have to follow the procedure for
choking (see pp. 66–73).

✤ **Care must be taken** when performing this
technique. Deaths have occurred where obstructions in the airway have been blown deeper into the
lungs.

GIVING ARTIFICIAL RESUSCITATION

1 Check the pulse (see p. 5). **2** If there is no heartbeat start chest compression (see pp. 9–12). **3** If there is a pulse clear the mouth of foreign material (see p. 4). **4** Push the chin up with one hand and tilt back the head. **5** Pinch the nose closed (**a**). **6** Take a deep breath, open your mouth wide and seal it around the victim's mouth (**b**). **7** Blow strongly into the mouth while watching for the chest to rise (**c**). **8** Once the chest has risen, ▶

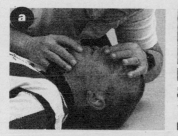

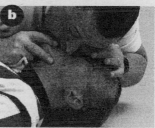

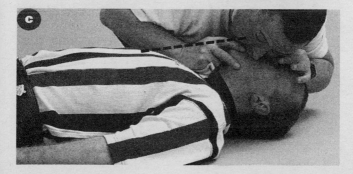

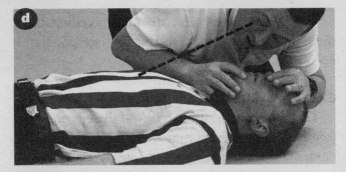

turn your head to watch the chest fall (**d**); finish breathing out. Give the first four breaths quickly. **9** Check the pulse. **10** Repeat actions 5 to 9 until the victim starts to breathe again.

An alternative to mouth-to-mouth resuscitation (if, for some reason, it is impossible) is mouth-to-nose. Close or cover the mouth firmly and blow into the nose, ensuring a good seal.

◆ **If the chest does not rise,** make the following checks.

CHECKS

1 That the nose is properly closed. **2** That the seal around the mouth or nose is tight. **3** That you are blowing hard enough.

◆ If, in spite of all, you are not succeeding, then there must be an airway obstruction (see pp. 4 and 66–73 for action).

EXTERNAL CHEST COMPRESSION

This is the procedure to follow if there is no pulse (see pp. 5–6). Chest compression used to be called "external cardiac massage" which was never a very accurate term. The heart cannot be massaged from the outside but it can be compressed.

POSITION OF THE HEART

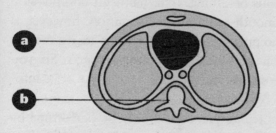

The heart (**a**) fills most of the space in the center of the chest between the breastbone in front and the spine (**b**), and surrounding muscles, behind. Because the front of the chest wall is normally quite mobile, it is possible to push back the breast bone and ribs a little and flatten the heart against the spine. The heart contains valves that allow the blood to pass in one direction only. Any compression of the heart forces the blood to move around the circulation in exactly the same way it does when the heart is contracting (beating) spontaneously.

Although hard work, it is perfectly possible to keep the circulation going by this kind of external compression. So long as air is, at the same time, being forced into the lungs, there is a good chance that the skin will regain its healthy color, the dilated pupils of the eyes will constrict, and that other signs of apparent recovery will occur (see p. 13). If the victim is capable of recovering, this procedure will often restart the spontaneous heartbeat and restore spontaneous breathing. External heart compression without mouth-to-mouth resuscitation, however, is futile. The purpose of the exercise is to restore the circulation of blood containing oxygen. So you must also supply the oxygen.

✤ **This technique should only be performed** by someone who is a trained first aider. The heartbeat must have completely stopped before external chest compression is given; otherwise, a faintly beating heart may be stopped by this procedure.

✤ **The following procedure,** for when only one person is present, should be performed by a trained first aider.

PERFORMING EXTERNAL CHEST COMPRESSION

1 Lay the victim flat on his back and kneel alongside. **2** Feel for the angle of the ribs at the bottom of the chest (**a**). Put the heel of one hand on the breastbone, two finger-breadths above the angle. **3** Cover your hand with your other hand. The thumbs and fingers should be kept raised. Lean forward so that your shoulders are above the breastbone. Keep your ▶

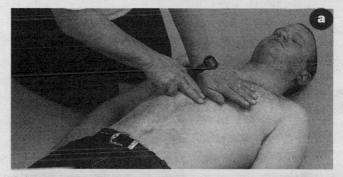

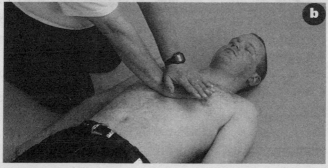

arms straight (**b**). **4** Press vertically down (**c**), depressing the front chest wall by 4–5 cm (1½–2 in). This is the dis-

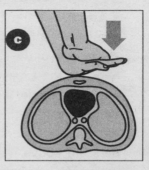

tance for an adult. Move the wall 2.5–4 cm (1–1½ in) for a child. Compress the chest in this way 15 times, at a rate that is faster than one push per second. Time the compressions by counting "one, two, three" quickly, compressing on each "one." **5** Move to the victim's head and give him two effective mouth-to-mouth puffs

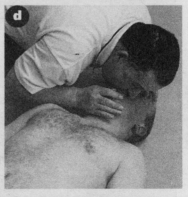

(**d**) to get air into the lungs (see p. 7). **6** Remember to watch the chest movements. **7** Repeat the cycle of 15 compressions and two lung inflations until the victim shows signs of recovery, until help arrives or until you are exhausted. **8** Check the pulse in the neck (see pp. 5–6) every 3 minutes.

SIGNS OF RECOVERY

- The blue, gray or purplish skin color disappears and the skin regains its healthy color.

- The pulse returns.

- The victim may groan or move.

- Spontaneous breathing returns and you feel resistance when performing artificial resuscitation.

RESUSCITATION BY TWO PEOPLE

Resuscitation by two people is much less exhausting than it is for one and can be continued longer. It is also more efficient because a better ratio of lung inflation to chest compression is possible. One inflation (see pp. 7–8) is given after every five chest compressions (see pp. 11–12). One person takes charge and this person supervises the airway, performs the mouth-to-mouth ventilation and checks the pulse. If the procedure is greatly prolonged the two people can switch over at intervals.

✤ **Timing is essential.** Do not attempt to inflate the chest while it is being compressed by the other person.

PERFORMING RESUSCITATION

1 The first person should ensure that the airway is clear, and establish that there is no breathing. **2** Start with two inflations (**a**). **3** Check the pulse. **4** The second person gives five chest compressions (**b**). **5** Give one inflation every time the fifth compression is released. **6** Repeat steps 4 and 5 until the victim starts to recover or until professional help arrives. **7** Check the neck pulse every two minutes (**c**).

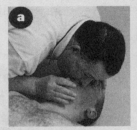

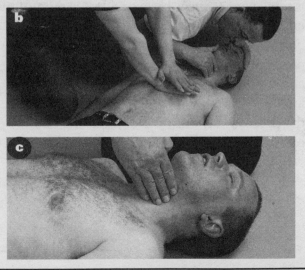

THE RECOVERY POSITION

When unconscious or semi-conscious people are left lying on their backs, they are in serious danger. This is because the muscles are relaxed and the normal reflexes that ensure an open and clear airway may not operate. The recovery position is used to avoid the dangers that can occur during unconsciousness.

DANGERS OF UNCONSCIOUSNESS

- The tongue may fall back to obstruct the throat and cut off the supply of air.

- Material of any kind, such as blood or vomit, may enter the air passages, because the opening to the larynx may not close automatically on contact with foreign matter, as it should.

- Such material may be inhaled, further obstructing the airway, causing a severe and dangerous form of pneumonia.

Unnecessary deaths occur in this way for want of a little knowledge, for example, the deaths of severely drunk people left lying on their backs.

✤ **Do not use the recovery position** if there is a risk of a spinal injury or if the casualty is not unconscious and is not likely to become so. However, if the airway is blocked, it must be cleared immediately. If an unconscious person must remain on his or her back, constantly check the airway.

PUTTING A PERSON IN
THE RECOVERY POSITION

1 Kneel to one side of the victim. **2** Place the arm nearest to you at right angles (**a**). **3** Bring the arm farthest from you across the chest, holding the palm of this arm against the ▶

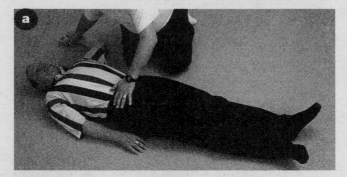

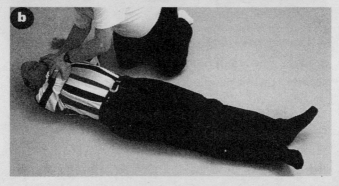

victim's cheek nearest you (**b**). **4** Holding the palm against the victim's cheek, raise the knee farthest from you (**c**). **5** Gently pull on the knee, turning the casualty toward you (**d**). ▶

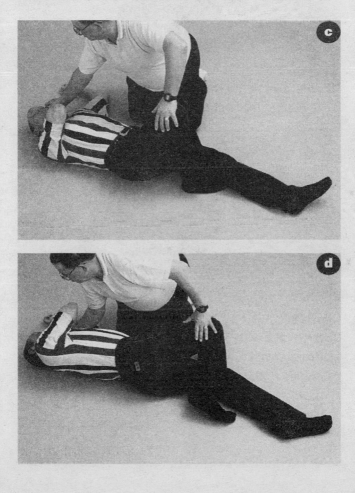

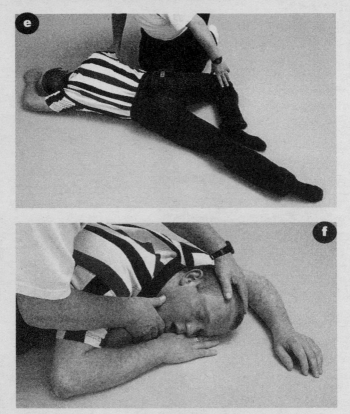

6 On the side to which the victim's head is turned, make sure the knee remains at right angles to the body (**e**). **7** Gently push the head back to ensure a clear airway and check the breathing (**f**).

♣ **Do not leave** the victim unattended.

SEVERE BLEEDING AND PRESSURE POINTS

In desperate cases, where severe bleeding continues, in spite of direct pressure by a pad or a bandage (see pp. 62–64) being applied to the wound, the flow of arterial blood may have to be stopped for a while but only as a last resort. By using indirect pressure on the artery leading to the wound, at the point where it runs over a bone, a life might be saved. The artery needs to be compressed between the fingers and the bone. In practice, indirect pressure can only be used to compress the main artery of the arm and the main artery of the leg. If effective, the procedure cuts off the whole blood supply to the limb.

PRESSURE POINTS

The main arm artery runs down the inner side of the upper arm bone (a), and is best compressed about the middle of the bone.

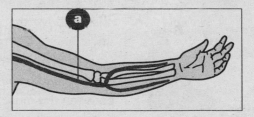

The main leg artery enters the leg at about the middle of the fold of the groin. At this point, it runs over a bony ridge on the pelvis (**b**), where it is best to apply the pressure.

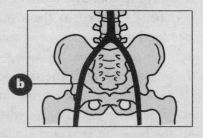

✤ **Do not cut off arterial blood supply** for more than 15 minutes at a time, otherwise there is danger of death (gangrene) of healthy tissue beyond the point of pressure.

✤ **Never use tourniquets.**

STOPPING ARM BLEEDING

1 Hold the injured arm so the hand is raised above the victim's head. **2** Press your fingertips firmly inwards and upwards between the muscles, on the inside of the upper arm, until you can feel the bone (**a**) and see that the bleeding is greatly reduced.

STOPPING LEG BLEEDING

1 The victim should be lying down with the knees slightly bent. **2** You must press the artery firmly against the pelvic bone with the heel of your hand or, if you are sure of

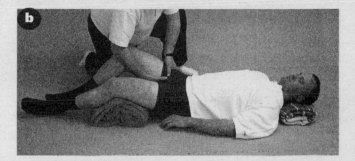

the location, with your thumbs (**b**). Strong pressure is necessary to compress this large artery.

2

Emergency Management of Serious Injuries

Principles and Responsibilities

THE JOB OF THE FIRST AIDER

The priorities, in order, are:

- always avoid endangering yourself;

- ensure that the victim is safe from danger, by moving him or her if necessary (see pp. 30–49);

- check the victim's condition and assess his or her injuries;

- take immediate remedial action if necessary.

♣ **Do not try to do too much:** remember that ambulance paramedics will know more than the lay first aider.

♣ **Do not attempt a precise diagnosis** of the victim's condition. Such a diagnosis will be made by a qualified doctor once the victim has been admitted to hospital.

✤ **Do not put on unnecessary bandages** or hold things up by treating trivial conditions. Give only essential first aid.

IMMEDIATE ACTION IN AN EMERGENCY

The first aider must, as quickly as possible, assess whether the injured person is either in immediate danger of dying or if his or her condition is likely to worsen.

CHECKING THE VICTIM'S CONDITION

Check **1** that there is no obstruction of the airway (**a**) (see p. 4); **2** that the victim is breath-

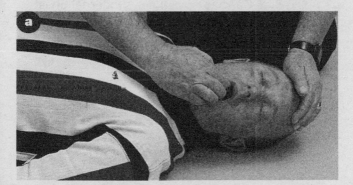

ing (**b**) (see p. 2); **3** that there is a pulse (**c**) (see p. 5)—to make sure cardiac arrest has not ▶

occurred; **4** for severe bleeding; **5** for shock (see pp. 104–108).

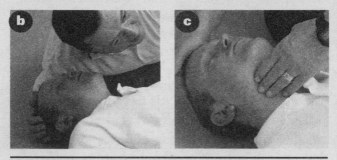

TAKING REMEDIAL ACTION

1 A blocked airway: see "Opening the airway," p. 3. **2** Air supply: see "Checking for breathing," p. 2, and "Artificial resuscitation," pp. 7–8. **3** Cardiac arrest: see "External chest compression," pp. 9–12. **4** Severe bleeding: see "Severe bleeding and pressure points," pp. 19–21. **5** Shock: see pp. 104–108. **6** Ask someone else (if possible) to call an ambulance (see p. 27) as soon as you have confirmed that the victim is not in danger of dying or that his or her condition is worsening. If you are alone with the victim and there is a good chance of someone else turning up, then you should stay to maintain the checks. **7** Reassure the victim. Remain calm at all times, and do whatever possible to reassure a conscious injured person that he or she will soon be properly looked after and on the way to recovery.

◆ **If there is little chance** of anyone else turning up, you must do what you can to safeguard the victim, and go for help.

✤ **Do not allow the victim to eat or drink,** except in the case of people with severe burns, who must be given sips of water.

✤ **Never move an injured person** unless it is absolutely necessary.

✤ **Do not be panicked** by noisy or hysterical behavior into thinking that a person must be gravely injured. Loud complainers are likely to be in a less serious condition than people lying quietly.

✤ **Avoid increasing the likelihood of shock** (see pp. 104–108).

SPECIFIC INJURIES AND CONDITIONS
BURNS AND SCALDS

Minimize the damage from burns and scalds by removing burning clothing and cooling the burned parts as quickly as possible with water (see pp. 84–85). Hot, wet clothing may continue to burn and should be dowsed with water before removal.

✤ **Do not remove burned clothing** if it has adhered to the victim's skin.

WOUND INFECTION

Open wounds must be covered in order to reduce the risk of wound infection (see pp. 151–152).

UNCONSCIOUS VICTIM

The airway of an unconscious victim must be safeguarded (see pp. 3–4).

FRACTURES

Further damage from broken bones (fractures) must be prevented by immobilizing the affected limb, so that movement at the fracture site is minimized, and further tissue injury avoided (see pp. 120–132).

✤ **Avoid using improvised splints** if an ambulance is on its way: ambulance paramedics will have better equipment for splinting fractures.

BODY TEMPERATURE

Wrap the victim in a blanket in order to maintain his or her body temperature.

✤ **Do not allow the victim to get too hot** by wrapping him or her up in too many layers or by using a hot-water bottle—this may cause skin flushing, because of widened blood vessels, and precipitate shock.

**WHAT THE EMERGENCY SERVICES
NEED TO KNOW**

First aiders or their assistants, after having dialed 911 and asked for the appropriate service, must pass on the following essential information.

<u>ESSENTIAL INFORMATION</u>

- The number from which they are calling—if the system doesn't already tell the dispatcher, so that they can be contacted again if necessary.

- The exact location or address of the incident. Local road names, proximity to road junctions or conspicuous landmarks all help to speed response time.

- The nature of the incident, its severity and its seeming degree of urgency.

- The nature of the injuries or illnesses.

- The number, age and sex of people injured.

- Any known hazards, e.g., gas, electric, chemical.

The HIV risk

It is necessary today to consider the possibility that an injured and bleeding person may be HIV positive and may offer a risk of infection to someone providing first aid. This risk is smaller than commonly supposed, as the following examples show.

EXAMPLES

- Very few medical and paramedical people have been infected by victims who are HIV positive. In those cases where infection has occurred, it has been transmitted via cuts or punctures which have become contaminated by the victim's infected blood.

- Surgeons engaged in operations on victims from areas of high AIDS prevalence, have, in about eight percent of cases, had direct skin contact with infected blood. Only a tiny number of these, however, have actually become infected themselves.

It is unlikely that a victim receiving first aid is HIV positive, and even if he or she is, the chances of a first aider actually acquiring the infection from such a person are very small.

Nevertheless, because the consequences of HIV infection are so serious, certain elementary precautions must always be taken.

PRECAUTIONS

- Spilled blood or other bodily fluids should be assumed to be infected, and it is strongly advised that contact with these should be avoided, if possible. There is a small but real danger of infection if HIV-positive blood contaminates cuts or abrasions possessed by a first aider.

• If the skin of a first aider comes into contact with a large quantity of the victim's blood, then the blood should be wiped away and the skin washed at the earliest possible opportunity. The risk of being infected in this way is, however, very small.

AVOIDING HIV INFECTION
WHEN THERE ARE FACIAL INJURIES

1 Cut a small slit in a thin plastic bag. **2** Place the bag on the victim's face, so that the slit is over the victim's mouth. This will enable mouth-to-mouth artificial respiration to take place without the first aider's mouth coming into skin-to-skin contact with that of the victim.

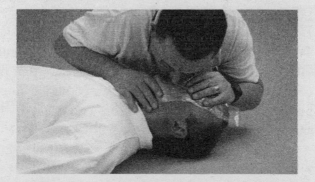

3 Perform artificial ventilation (see pp. 7–8) by blowing through the slit.

- First aiders must try to avoid getting blood in their eyes: though the risk is small, HIV infection can occur through the membrane that covers the whites of the eyes (the conjunctiva). Any visible blood should be washed out.

- The risk from saliva contamination during mouth-to-mouth artificial resuscitation (see pp. 7–8) is believed to be negligible. It is probably a little greater, however, if there is bleeding around the victim's mouth. In this situation, it is necessary to give the victim's mouth a quick clean before starting. If the risk still seems real, then the procedure shown on p. 29 can be used.

Moving and Lifting Victims

The primary considerations for the first aider are to safeguard the victim's wellbeing and ensure that he or she is comfortable. The victim's condition must not be aggravated, nor their life endangered, by careless handling.

WHEN TO MOVE AN INJURED PERSON

An injured person should be moved only when medical help is not readily available, or when there is immediate danger to life. The following are examples of situations where it may be necessary to move victims.

EXAMPLES

- On a busy road which cannot be blocked off.

- In a dangerous building, perhaps threatened by fire or possibility of collapse.

- In a building containing gas or poisonous fumes, such as a garage full of carbon monoxide (see p. 76).

BEFORE YOU MOVE AN INJURED PERSON

- If it is necessary to move the victim, then try first to assess the nature and severity of the injuries, especially to the neck or spine. Examine the head and neck, chest and abdomen, and all limbs which, if injured, must be supported during removal.

- If there is any doubt about the severity of injuries in an injured (but conscious and freely breathing) person who has to be moved, then aim to move the victim in exactly the position in which he or she was found.

♣ **Avoid moving a person** with a severe crush injury—it may do great harm (see pp. 108–111).

✤ **Single first aiders** should never attempt to move victims by themselves when help is available.

GENERAL RULES FOR LIFTING

The following principles should always be adhered to in all cases where victims have to be lifted.

PRINCIPLES

A first aider must:

- get close to the victim;

- keep the feet comfortably apart, to ensure a firm stance and a stable, balanced posture;

- lower him- or herself to the victim's level by bending the knees, not the back (a);

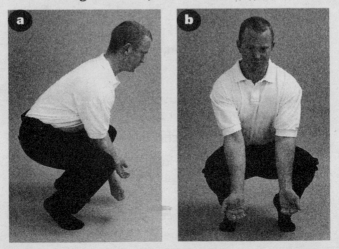

- keep the back straight (**b**);

- grasp the victim firmly, using the whole hand;

- lift with the legs, not the back, and use the shoulders to support the weight of the victim.

◆ **If the victim begins to slip**, let him or her slide gently to the ground, to avoid causing further injury.

✤ **Do not try to prevent** the casualty from falling: this may lead to injury to your back.

✤ **Do not try to lift** too heavy a weight—get assistance whenever possible: the larger the group of people lifting the victim, the smaller the chances of causing or incurring injury.

WHICH METHOD TO USE

Various methods are used to move or lift injured persons. The method to be used in any particular situation depends on the following points:

- the number of available helpers;

- the size and weight of the victim;

- the distance the victim has to be carried;

- the terrain across which the victim has to be moved;

- the type and the severity of the injury sustained by the victim;

- the equipment and amenities available to the first aider.

ONE FIRST AIDER

DRAGGING THE VICTIM

This method should only be used when the victim cannot be lifted, is not capable of standing up, and has to be moved quickly. It is performed in the following way.

---

1 Fold the victim's arms across the chest (**a**).
2 Pull back the victim's unbuttoned overcoat ▶

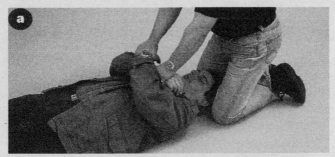

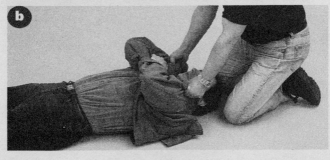

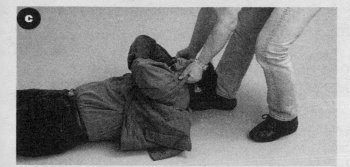

or jacket and place it underneath the head (**b**).
3 Crouch down behind the victim, grasp the
shoulders of the clothing, and tug the victim
smoothly away (**c**).

◆ If the victim
is not wearing a
jacket or an over-
coat, then you
must hold the
victim underneath
the armpits and
tug.

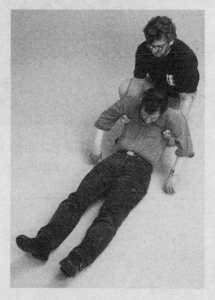

THE HUMAN CRUTCH

This method can be used when a victim can walk but requires assistance.

---

1 Stand at the victim's injured side. **2** Place the victim's arm around your neck and hold

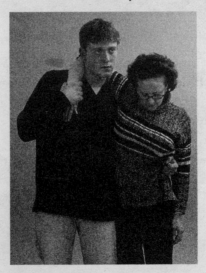

the victim's hand. **3** Put the other arm around the victim's waist, grasping the clothing at the hip.

✚ **Do not use this method** if the victim has received an injury to the upper limbs.

THE CRADLE

This method is suitable for children or victims who are not heavy.

Carry the victim by placing one arm under the thighs, and the other above the waist.

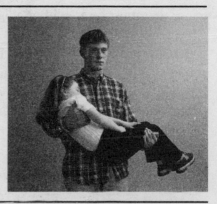

PIGGYBACK

A small, light and conscious victim, who is strong enough to hold on to a first aider, may be carried in piggyback fashion.

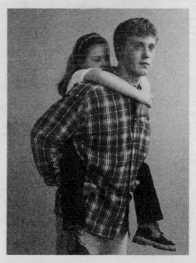

THE FIREMAN'S LIFT

This method can be used when the first aider requires a free hand and if the victim must be moved. The victim can be conscious or unconscious, but must be a child or a lightweight adult.

---

1 Help the victim to stand. **2** Take hold of the victim's right wrist with your left hand (**a**). **3** Bend your knees, bend forward, and carefully put your right shoulder into the victim's groin, letting the victim fall gently across ▸

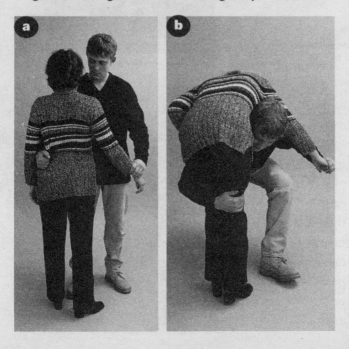

your shoulders.
4 Put your right
arm around and
behind the victim's
knees (**b**). **5** Stand
up and adjust the
victim's weight
across your shoul-
ders (**c**).

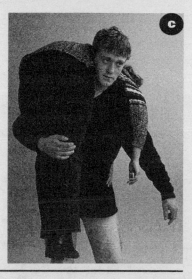

◆ If the victim
cannot stand, he
or she must be
turned face-down,
if necessary, and
pulled up on to his
or her knees and
then into a stand-
ing position. Stand
close and lift by
passing your arms
under the victim's
armpits.

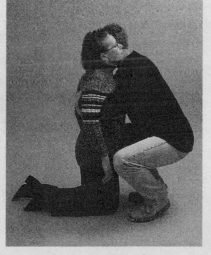

TWO FIRST AIDERS

Two people, lifting together, can provide a carrier seat for a victim.

THE FOUR-HANDED SEAT

This method is used when the victim is in a condition to use one or both arms to assist the first aiders.

---

1 Each person grasps his or her own left wrist with the right hand, and then the other's right wrist with the left hand (**a**).

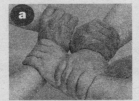

2 Both squat down. **3** The victim sits on their hands and puts an arm around each person's neck (**b**).
4 Both carriers rise together.
5 The carriers step out simultaneously, stepping first with their outside feet, and walk forward at an ordinary pace.

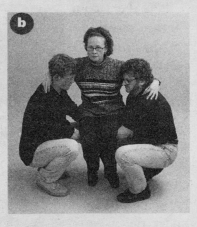

THE TWO-HANDED SEAT

This seat is used to transport a victim who is unable to assist the first aiders, usually because of injury to the arms.

---

1 Two first aiders squat facing each other on either side of the victim. **2** They pass the fore-

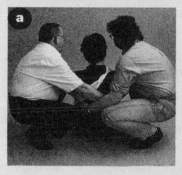

arms nearest to the victim's body under the victim's back, just below the shoulders, and grasp the victim's clothing (**a**). **3** The first-aiders slightly raise the victim's

back, pass their other arms under the middle of the victim's thighs and grasp each other's wrists (**b**). **4** The first aiders rise simultaneously, start walking using the feet on the outside, and continue at an ordinary pace.

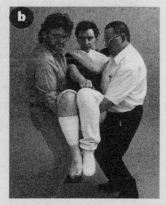

◆ If there is no clothing for the first aiders to grasp, then they must, if possible, grasp each other's wrists.

THE KITCHEN CHAIR METHOD

When a victim has to be moved along passageways, or up and down stairs, the kitchen chair method is most suitable. The victim must be conscious and must not have serious injuries.

---

1 Test the chair to ensure that it can comfortably carry the victim's weight. **2** Ensure that the way is cleared of all obstructions, such as loose carpeting. **3** Secure the trunk and thighs of the victim to the chair with scarves or large

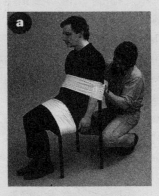

bandages (**a**). **4** First aiders should stand at the front and rear of the chair, and tilt it backwards (to an angle of about 30° from the horizontal) before lifting it (**b**). **5** One first aider supports the back of the chair and the victim; the other (who is facing the victim) holds the chair by its front legs and moves carefully ◗

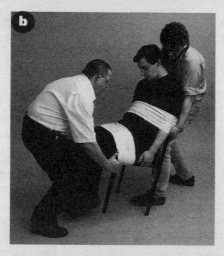

backwards down the stairs or along the passageway.

◆ **If the stairs or passageway** are sufficiently
wide, the first aiders can stand by the sides of the
chair, each holding one back and one front chair leg.

❖ **Never tilt the chair** without previously inform-
ing the victim: neglecting to do so risks causing the
victim further injury and distress.

STRETCHERS

Stretchers are useful for moving victims over long
distances. In the event of no stretcher being available, you can make an improvised one. As a general
rule, try always to ensure, when using a stretcher,

that the position of the victim's head and neck is aligned with his or her body, and make sure that the airway is unobstructed.

◆ **If a blanket is available,** it should be draped across the stretcher before the victim is placed on it. Wrap it around the victim when he or she has been placed on the stretcher.

◆ **If strong jackets or coats are not available,** then try the substitutes listed below.

- Strong sacks: make holes in the bottom corners of one or more sacks. Pass the poles through them.

- Broad bandages: these can be firmly tied, at intervals, to two poles.

- A strong blanket, tarpaulin, rug or piece of sacking: spread the material out, lay the poles in place and fold the material over from both sides so that the weight of the victim keeps it in place.

MAKING AN IMPROVISED STRETCHER

1 Find two or three strong jackets or coats.
2 Turn the sleeves of the coats inside out and pass a strong pole (such as a broomstick) through one of the sleeves of each jacket (**a**),

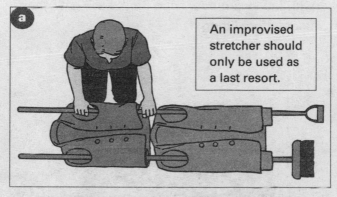

An improvised stretcher should only be used as a last resort.

and a second pole through the others. **3** Button or zip up the jackets to complete the stretcher (**b**). **4** Test the stretcher, if possible, by getting an uninjured person to lie on it, and then lift it to ensure that it can safely handle the weight.

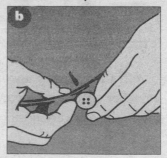

MOVING A VICTIM ONTO A STRETCHER

1 One first aider must carefully roll the victim on to the uninjured side. **2** The other first aider must then place the open stretcher flat against the victim's back. **3** Carefully roll the stretcher, with the victim now lying on it, back onto the floor before lifting it up.

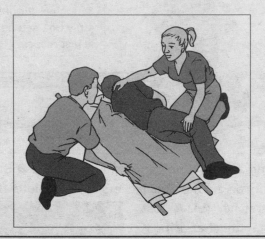

◆ **If the victim is unconscious,** position the open stretcher against the victim's front, and carry him or her in the recovery position (see pp. 16–18).

MORE THAN TWO FIRST AIDERS
TURNING A VICTIM WITH SUSPECTED SPINE INJURY

It is necessary to turn such a victim on to his or her side when he or she is vomiting, to ensure that the victim does not choke on his or her own vomit, and to avoid any distress or discomfort which could cause them to move, and possibly further exacerbate the injury.

Six people are required to perform this task.

Three people must hold the victim on one side, two on the other and one at the head. Turn the victim very carefully, without any twisting or bending of the spine.

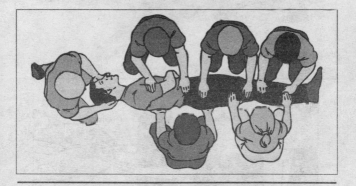

✤ Never ever allow the victim's head to move out of alignment with their body.

MOVING A VICTIM WITH SUSPECTED
SPINE FRACTURE

Seven people are required to make such a removal.

---

1 Firmly hold the victim's head, shoulders and pelvis and place pads of soft material between the ankles, knees and thighs **(a)**. **2** Tie the ▶

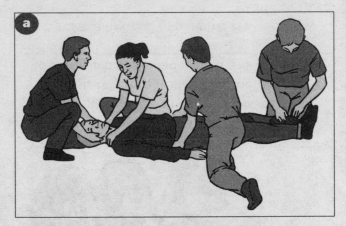

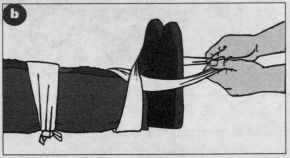

victim's legs together. The feet should be tied together with a figure-eight bandage (see p. 190) (**b**; see opposite page). **3** Position three people on each side of the victim. **4** The remaining first aider must then squat at the head of the victim (looking down the axis of the victim's body), and keep the victim's head and neck aligned; this is achieved by carefully placing a hand on either side of the victim's head. The person at the head gives the orders to the lifters. **5** Roll the victim slightly, so that the lifters can get their arms under the victim's body (**c**).

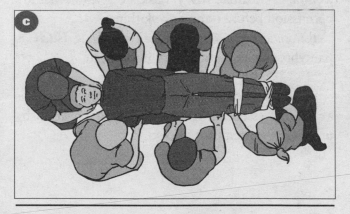

❖ **Never ever allow the victim's head** to move out of alignment with the body.

Removing Clothing and Helmets

REMOVING CLOTHING

It is sometimes necessary to remove clothing in order to perform proper treatment, reveal injuries or to obtain clues to the victim's condition.

Many injuries, however, can be inspected without having to resort to clothes removal: fractures can readily be found without removing clothing, and major wounds are likely to have occurred with obvious tearing of the clothing.

If clothing must be removed, then take off only the minimum amount and try to disturb the victim as little as possible. Always ask a conscious victim's permission before removing clothing.

Removal of a woman's underclothing (such as pantyhose) may be necessary if it is tight.

✤ **Never attempt to remove clothing** unless it is absolutely essential: much harm can be done by unnecessary attempts to do so.

REMOVING COATS, JACKETS, SHIRTS AND VESTS

1 Raise the victim and slip the garment over the shoulders (**a**). **2** Bend the arm on the victim's uninjured side and remove the garment. **3** Gently slip out the other arm (**b**).

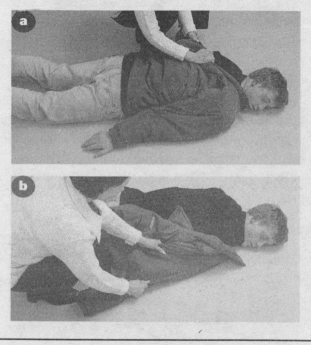

◆ **If removal is proving difficult,** then slitting the seam of the garment along the injured side may be helpful.

TROUSERS

1 Raise the trouser leg if the calf or knee is injured (**a**). **2** Pull the trousers down from the waist if the thigh is injured (**b**).

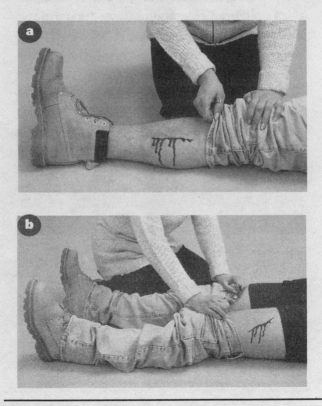

◆ **If removal is proving difficult,** then the first aider should slit the inner seam of the trouser leg.

REMOVING SHOES OR BOOTS

1 Steady the victim's ankle (**a**).

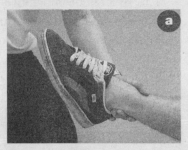

2 Cut or undo any laces (**b**).

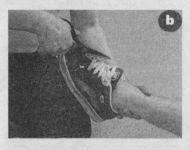

3 Remove the shoe (**c**).

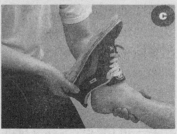

◆ **If there is difficulty** in removing long boots, then carefully slit them up the back seam with a razor blade or sharp knife.

REMOVING SOCKS

The first aider must use the following method only when having difficulty in removing socks in the ordinary way.

1 Two fingers must be inserted between the sock and the victim's leg. **2** The edge of the sock must be raised and then cut between the first aider's fingers.

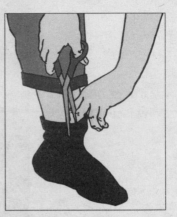

REMOVING HELMETS

The removal of two types of helmet—protective helmets and full-face crash helmets—is described here. First aiders are, in general, strongly advised not to try to remove a helmet, as such an action may—in the event of a neck fracture—cause paralysis or even death. In most cases, severe head injuries are actually prevented by crash helmets. If a helmet (of whatever type) has to be removed, remember the following points:

- take off any eyeglasses or sunglasses before removal;

- it is always best if the victim can remove the helmet him- or herself, if possible.

REMOVING A PROTECTIVE HELMET

A protective helmet is here defined as that type which only covers the wearer's head.

---

1 Unfasten or cut the chin strap (**a**).
2 A second person should support the victim's head and neck.
3 Force the sides of the helmet apart.
4 Lift the helmet up and back (**b**).

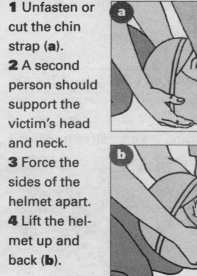

REMOVING A FULL-FACE CRASH HELMET

Two people are required for this operation: one to support the victim's neck and head; the other to remove the helmet.

❖ **A full-face crash helmet should never be removed unless it is a matter of life and death. Remove the helmet only if:**

- the victim's breathing is hampered by the helmet;

- the victim is not breathing and has no pulse;

- the victim is vomiting.

---

1 Place your hands on each side of the helmet. Keep the head steady by placing your fingers on the victim's jaw. **2** A second person should cut or loosen the chin strap (**a**). **3** He ▶

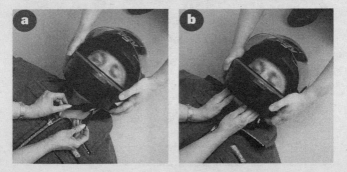

or she should then support the victim's head by holding it at the base of the skull and the jawbone (**b**). **4** Tilt the helmet back to clear the chin and nose (**c**). **5** Tilt it forward to clear the base of the victim's skull (**d**). **6** Lift off the helmet (**e**).

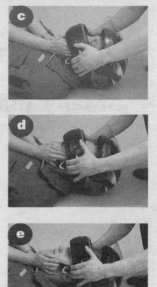

3

Major Injuries and Dangerous Conditions

Bleeding

WOUNDS AND EXTERNAL BLEEDING

<u>MINOR WOUNDS</u>

See pp. 149–152 for the treatment and management of minor wounds.

Abrasions (a). These are on the surface only and are caused by a grazing or scraping. Bleeding is minimal.

Contusions (b). These are on and just under the surface, with skin splitting and bruising. Bleeding is seldom severe.

<u>MAJOR WOUNDS</u>

Incised wounds (c). These are cleanly cut by a

TYPES OF WOUND

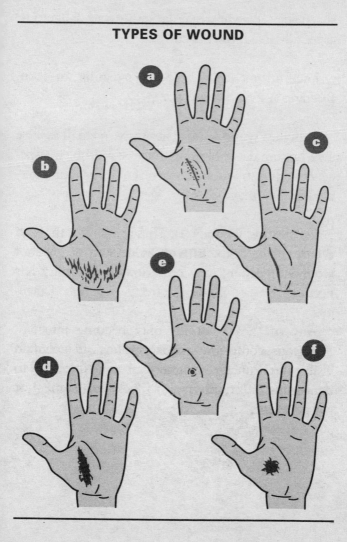

sharp edge. Bleeding may be severe and dangerous, especially if an artery is cut.

Lacerations (d). These are irregular or torn. Bleeding is sometimes severe.

Puncture wounds (e). These have a small surface area but are deep. Bleeding may be a problem especially with stab wounds, when serious or fatal internal bleeding may occur.

Perforating wounds (f). These pass right through a part of the body, as with some stab or gunshot wounds. Bleeding may be serious if an artery has been cut.

Any of these wounds may become infected. Abrasions, contusions and lacerations often contain visible dirt. Puncture wounds can sometimes lead to dangerous infections, such as lockjaw (tetanus) or gas gangrene.

<u>BLOOD LOSS AND ITS CONTROL</u>

The whole body contains about 5 liters (9 pints) of blood. If an artery is cut, the blood is pumped out under pressure with each heartbeat and can usually be seen to be spurting in time with the pulse. Blood from an artery is bright red; blood from a vein is a dull purplish color.

Minor bleeding. This often comes from the blood capillaries and is usually an ooze or a trickle. Such bleeding offers no significant risk.

Arterial bleeding. This is one of the few real emergencies with which the first aider must deal. If unchecked, it may soon lead to so much blood loss that the circulation cannot be maintained (shock, see pp. 104–108), also fatally depriving the brain and heart muscle of blood. Torn arteries often bleed less profusely than cleanly cut vessels.

The only thing that takes priority over stopping arterial bleeding is ensuring that the victim is breathing freely. As soon as you see arterial bleeding apply direct pressure to the affected part.

Bleeding from veins. This is not pulsatile and is usually less serious but blood can gush if a large vein, such as a major varicose vein or one of the main internal veins, is injured.

CONTROLLING BLEEDING

1 Apply direct pressure to the wound, using your fingers or hand (**a**). **2** If the wound is large, press the edges together, gently and firmly maintaining pressure (**b**). **3** Consider what you can use as a pad to control the bleeding more effectively. A clean folded handkerchief is often ideal. **4** If bleeding is from a limb, elevate it (**c**). ▶

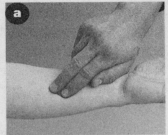

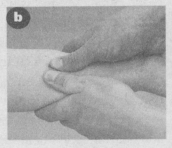

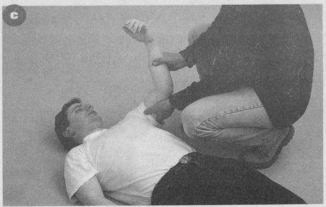

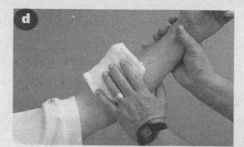

Be careful if there
is a possibility of a
fracture (see pp.
121–123). **5** If direct
pressure seems to

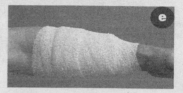

be controlling the bleeding and you have a
first aid kit, put a sterile or clean dressing (see
pp. 173–176) on the wound, covering it completely. **6** Apply a pad (see p. 176) that covers
the area of the wound. Press it down firmly
(**d**). **7** Bandage it securely in place (**e**).

✤ **The bandage should be firm enough** to prevent bleeding but not so tight as to cut off the circulation altogether. To check the circulation, find a
pulse or press a nail of the injured limb until it turns
white. When the pressure is released, the nail should
become pink. If the circulation is affected, the nail
will remain white or blue; and the extremities will
feel very cold. Also, if it is the arm that is injured,

check the wrist pulse (see p. 5) to see if blood is continuing to circulate.

◆ **If there is still bleeding** from under the pad, do not remove it. This will disturb any clot that has formed and make the bleeding worse. Just put another large pad on top and bandage firmly.

◆ **If the bleeding still will not stop** and is severe after using direct pressure or bandaging, you will have to use pressure on the artery leading to the wound (see "Severe bleeding and pressure points," pp. 19–21).

<u>FOREIGN BODIES IN WOUNDS</u>

Although dirt and other loose small-particle foreign material should be carefully washed out of minor wounds, larger foreign bodies should be left alone.

✤ **Never** try to pry foreign bodies out of deep wounds. This may precipitate severe bleeding.

MANAGING WOUNDS WITH
FOREIGN BODIES

Control bleeding and, if bleeding is not severe, dress the wound as for an open fracture (see pp. 124–127).

INTERNAL BLEEDING

This is often difficult to detect, but should be suspected when injuries are severe, as in traffic accidents or a thigh fracture.

FEATURES

- Bleeding from an orifice, such as the mouth, nose or ears.

- Growing swelling and tension.

- Extensive bruising.

- Restlessness.

- Signs of shock (see pp. 105–106).

IN THE EVENT OF INTERNAL BLEEDING

1 Call 911 immediately. The need to get the victim to a hospital is very great. **2** Check and record the pulse rate every 5 minutes. **3** Treat for shock (see pp. 104–108).

Breathing Difficulties

Minor breathing difficulty, such as mild asthma, will not require first aid but, unless the cause is known, medical advice should always be sought. Severe breathing difficulty is highly dangerous and calls for immediate remedial action. Airway obstruction (see pp. 3–4) is one of the most serious emergencies and it is one in which knowledgeable first aid, effectively applied, often can save a life.

ASPHYXIA

Asphyxia means lack of oxygen in the blood. It is caused by the interruption of the free flow of air into and out of the tiny air sacs in the lungs. This is usually the cause of death in choking (opposite), drowning (see pp. 74–75), strangulation (see pp. 78–79), inhalation of a gas or fumes which exclude oxygen (see pp. 76–78), foreign body airway obstruction (see pp. 3–4) and swelling of the soft tissues of the voice box (oedema of the larynx).

If asphyxia is being caused by any external agency, such as a plastic bag or a pillow, this should, of course, be removed at once and the breathing (see p. 2) and pulse (see p. 5) checked. Appropriate resuscitation, if necessary, should immediately be undertaken (see pp. 7–12).

CHOKING

Choking is commonly caused by the inhalation of a foreign body, such as a lump of ill-chewed food or a hard candy, into the voice box (larynx) or major air passages (a). This can happen if a person is laughing or starts to sneeze while eating. Airway obstruction of this kind cannot be helped by mouth-to-mouth ventilation—which might, indeed, make matters worse. The urgent necessity is to get rid of the obstruction, after which artificial resuscitation (see pp. 7–8) may be supplied, if necessary.

<u>FEATURES</u>

The victim

- grasps her throat (a highly characteristic sign) (**b**);

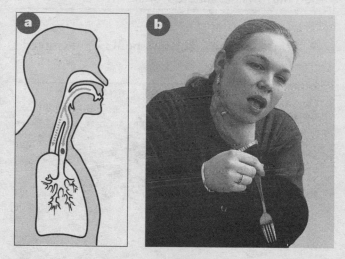

- shows marked indications of distress and panic;

- is unable to talk;

- may first breathe noisily then not at all;

- turns blue or sometimes gray or pale;

- becomes unconscious within a minute or so.

COUGHING UP THE OBSTRUCTION

Conscious adult and child. 1 If the victim is an adult, ask him or her if choking is occurring. **2** If air can be inhaled, encourage strong coughing after slow inhalation. Violent inhalation may make matters worse.

◆ If this fails, the following should be attempted.

BENDING AND SLAPPING

Conscious adult. 1 The victim should bend over so that the head is lower than the lungs. **2** Slap him sharply between the shoulder blades with the heel of the hand.

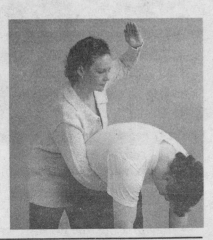

Do not be afraid of hurting him. This is a dire emergency and life is in danger.

Conscious child.
Rest him, face down, on your knees and try slapping between the shoulder blades with the heel of the hand. Try this four times if necessary.

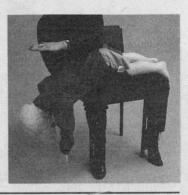

Unconscious adult and child. 1 Turn the victim onto the side closest to you. **2** Push the head back. **3** Slap the back four times, if necessary, with the heel of your hand.

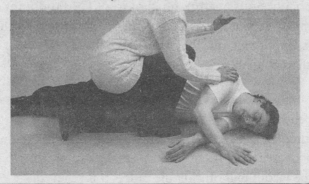

Babies and infants.
1 The infant should be supported, face down, on the forearm.
2 The head and chest should be supported by the hand. **3** Give the infant four smart slaps between the shoulder blades with your fingers.

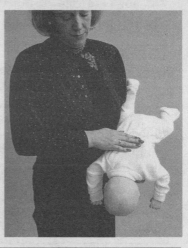

◆ **If this fails,** use the abdominal thrust method.

THE ABDOMINAL THRUST METHOD

This can be used either on a conscious or an unconscious victim of choking. The abdominal thrust should cause a sudden rise in pressure in the lungs, driving out the obstruction like a cork from a champagne bottle.

✤ **This should not be tried** unless coughing, and bending and slapping have failed, as it may cause internal injury. Do not, however, omit it on this account, for if there is complete airway obstruction, the victim will quickly die unless it is relieved.

USING THE ABDOMINAL THRUST

Conscious adult.

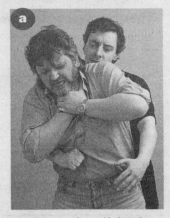

1 Stand behind him, put one arm around him, clench your fist and place it in the middle of the abdomen, between the navel and the lower angle of the ribs (**a**). **2** Turn the thumb inwards. **3** Grasp your fist with the other hand (**b**) and pull both firmly against the victim's body (**c**). **4** Suddenly, thrust inwards and upwards with considerable force so as to compress the upper ▶

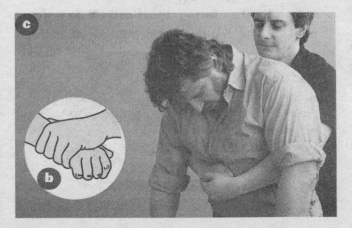

abdomen and push upwards on the diaphragm—the muscular sheet that is the flexible floor of the chest. **5** Repeat up to four times, if necessary.

Conscious child.
1 Take the child on your knee. **2** Thrust with one fist only, using counter-pressure on the back with the other hand.

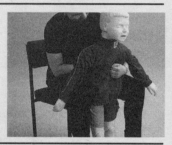

Unconscious adult. 1 Turn her on her back with the chin up and the head tilted back. **2** Kneel alongside or, preferably, astride the upper thighs, facing the head. **3** Put the heel of one hand on the midline of the ▸

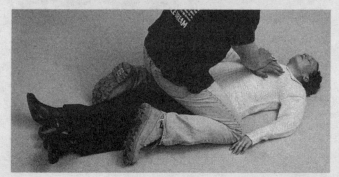

upper abdomen, between the navel and the rib angle, and cover it with your other hand. Thrust forcibly inwards and upwards.
4 Repeat up to four times.

Unconscious child. Perform the thrust as with adults but using one hand only.

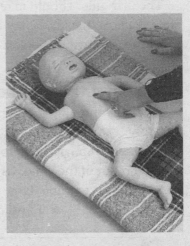

Babies and Infants. Whether conscious or unconscious, lay him or her down and perform the thrust with two fingers.

After a successful procedure on an unconscious person, clear out the mouth with hooked fingers (see p. 4), so that the obstruction is completely removed.

◆ If there is any residual breathing difficulty, call 911 even if the patient appears to have recovered, as swelling of the airway may occur.

DROWNING

Never assume that a person has drowned even if she has been under water for many minutes. People have recovered fully after immersion in cold water for half an hour. This is possible as body cooling slows metabolic processes and the brain can survive the lack of oxygen for longer than normal.

The first aider should take into account any possible dangers that they may encounter when trying to rescue a drowning person.

RESUSCITATING A DROWNING PERSON

1 While removing the person from the water, apply mouth-to-mouth ventilation (**a**). In between breaths, move to dry land. **2** Get the person out of the water as quickly as possible. **3** Check breathing (see p. 2). **4** Check the pulse (see p. 5). **5** If artifical resuscitation is ▶

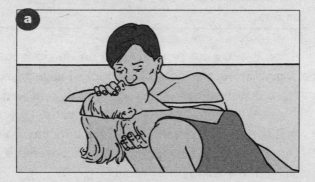

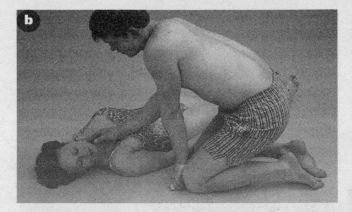

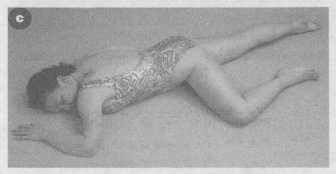

still needed, turn the victim's head to the side (**b**) and clear the mouth of any material (see p. 4). Also, the victim will bring up water. **6** If the victim is breathing, put her into the recovery position (**c**) (see pp. 16–18). **7** If the victim is breathing but is very cold, treat for hypothermia (see pp. 116–118). **8** Get the victim to a hospital as soon as possible.

FUMES AND GASES
CARBON MONOXIDE POISONING

This is a colorless, odorless, tasteless and poisonous gas, present in large quantity in the exhaust of motor vehicles. It is also produced by coal-burning fires or furnaces. Carbon monoxide combines readily with the hemoglobin of the blood, forming a stable compound (carboxyhemoglobin) and cutting the ability of the red blood cells to carry oxygen. If half an adult's hemoglobin becomes carboxyhemoglobin, this may lead to death.

Rapid rescue of a person, e.g., from a closed garage, is unlikely to be dangerous, especially if doors and windows are opened. Do not put yourself at risk.

ONCE THE VICTIM IS IN THE OPEN AIR

1 Check for breathing (**a**) (see p. 2). **2** Check ▶

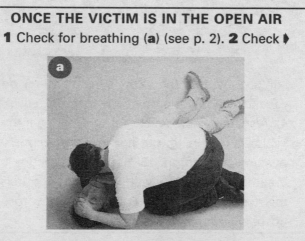

the pulse (see p. 5).
3 Perform resuscitation if needed (see pp. 7–8). **4** Put the victim into the recovery position (**b**) (see pp. 16–18). **5** Arrange for removal to a hospital.

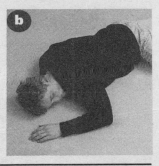

SMOKE INHALATION

The fire that causes smoke will reduce the local available oxygen, leading to asphyxia. Smoke is often highly irritating to the airway and may even cause tight closure of the vocal cords, thus cutting off the airway. Some types of smoke are very poisonous. You will need to decide whether to risk attempting an immediate removal of the victim, or victims, from the fire or whether first to call 911.

Once the victim has been dragged away from the smoke and their burning clothes have been dealt with (see p. 83), take the following measures.

IN THE EVENT OF SMOKE INHALATION

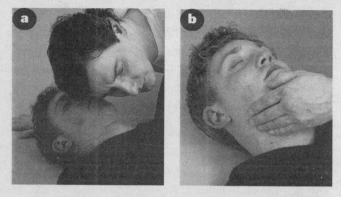

1 Check the airway, breathing (see p. 2) (**a**) and pulse (see p. 5) (**b**). **2** Perform artificial resuscitation if necessary (see pp. 7–8). **3** Check for burns and treat appropriately (see pp. 86–88 and 156–157). **4** Arrange for removal to a hospital.

STRANGULATION

Unconsciousness or death may result from compression of the arteries in the neck as well as from interference with the airway. There may also be spinal injury.

IN THE EVENT OF STRANGULATION

1 Relieve the constriction around the neck by lifting up and supporting the victim (**a**), so that the weight can be taken off the neck. **2** Cut the ligature beneath the knot (**b**). **3** Check for breathing (see p. 2). **4** Check the pulse (see p. 5). **5** Perform resuscitation, if needed (see pp. 7–8). **6** Place in the recovery position, if necessary. **7** Arrange for transport to a hospital.

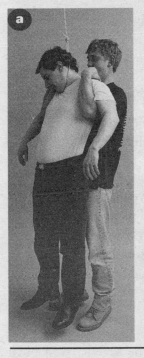

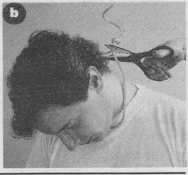

Contact the police on all occasions of discovering a strangulation. Keep all materials as evidence and, if possible, record the condition in which you found the victim.

Burns

CAUSES

Burns are tissue injuries caused by

- high or very low temperatures;

- radiation: sunlight and other ultraviolet sources, X-rays, gamma rays;

- corrosive chemicals;

- electrical current flowing through the body— this has a heating and coagulating effect and may interfere with breathing and the heartbeat;

- friction.

Tissue is liable to be destroyed if the causal agent is allowed to continue to act. First aid thus consists, if possible, of reducing (or raising) temperature, removing the victim from the source of radiation, or removing the injurious chemical by brushing and/or washing.

BURN DEPTH

Depth is an indication of the severity of a burn and determines whether treatment is necessary and, if so, what kind is needed. Burns are grouped by depth into three categories.

Superficial (a) These affect the surface layer only,

causing redness, swelling and tenderness. They normally heal well without leaving scars. Small superficial burns may not need medical attention.

Intermediate (b) These cause blisters and are liable to get infected.

Deep (c) These involve the full thickness of the skin. They appear gray, waxy-looking or charred, and may be painless, even if large, because the nerves may have been destroyed. Large burns will usually be in the deep category.

BURN DEPTH

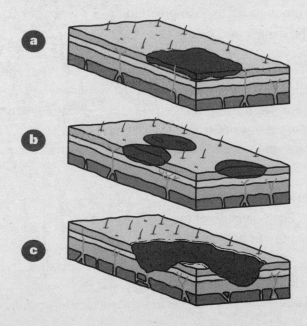

BURN AREA

The larger the area of the burn, the more serious it is likely to be. Even superficial burns can be dangerous if very large. Burns over 3 cm (1¼ in) across should be seen by a doctor. In large burns, an assessment of the danger is made using the "rule of nines." Any person with a burn, even a superficial burn, of more than 9 percent of the body area, will require hospital attention. Surgical shock (see pp. 104–108) and infection are the main risks to life from extensive burns; the rule of nines is an important way of assessing the danger and determining the need for blood or other transfusions. After the first 48 hours, the main danger is from infection.

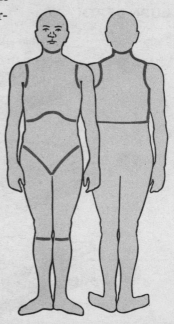

THE RULE OF NINES

Each division of the human body, shown here, represents 9 percent of its total surface area.

CLOTHING ON FIRE

Many serious burns are caused by clothing, especially loose, light clothing like nightgowns, catching fire. Fire starting at the hem often spreads rapidly upwards by convection, if the person concerned remains standing or runs about.

IF CLOTHING IS ON FIRE

1 Make the victim lie down at once. **2** Use a dry powder extinguisher if you have one, or try to smother the flames with any suitable heavy material. This will exclude oxygen. If no smothering materials are at hand lie the victim's burning side on the ground to extinguish the flames.

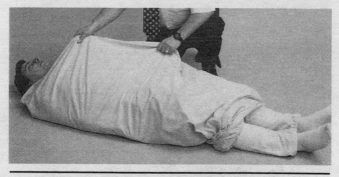

❖ Do not use nylon.

❖ Do not roll the person along the ground as this may extend the burned area.

ONCE THE FLAMES ARE OUT

Rapid cooling is the next priority. Do not waste any time.

RAPID COOLING AND PREVENTING INFECTION

1 Hot clothing can cause serious burns, so remove or cut them off or cool with water.
2 Cool the victim for the next 10 minutes by pouring buckets and jugs of cold water over him (**a**). **3** Call 911. **4** Check that the airway ▶

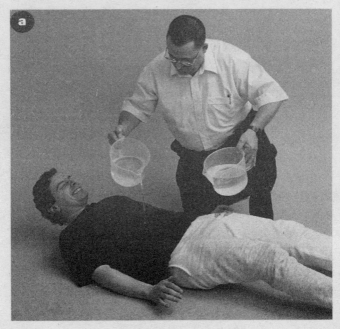

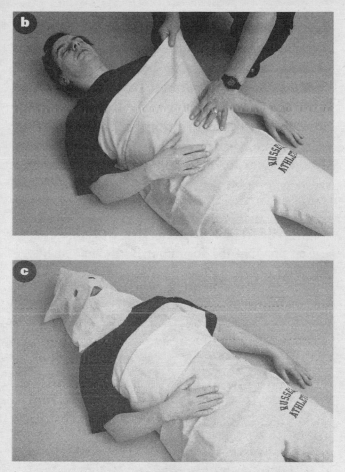

is clear (see pp. 2–4). **5** Cover the burns (**b, c**) with clean dressings to reduce the risk of infection. **6** Give the victim regular sips of cold water, if conscious, to replace any lost fluid.

HIGH-TEMPERATURE BURNS AND SCALDS

There is no essential difference between high-temperature burns and scalds; both are tissue injuries caused by high temperatures. Tissue damage occurs rapidly, and the most important thing that can be done is for the temperature of the burn to be reduced immediately. Cooling may greatly reduce the severity of the burn and will rapidly relieve the severe pain of burning.

TREATING BURNS AND SCALDS

See pp. 156–157 for minor burns and scalds.

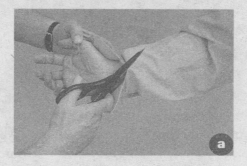

1 Remove or cut away any clothes that are covering the burned area (**a**). **2** Remove any potentially constricting objects (rings, bracelets, watches, etc.) before swelling occurs. **3** Hold the burned part under a cold tap, a garden hose or a cold shower, and run ▶

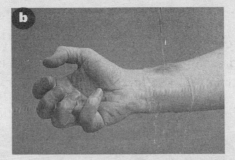

the water on it for at least 10 minutes (**b**). This measure alone can make the difference between a serious and a trivial burn and should be used, if possible, for all burns.

❖ **Do not apply** butter, ointments or lotions.
❖ **Do not pull** off anything that is stuck to a burn.

BLISTERS
These should be kept intact if at all possible. Blisters may be protected by careful padding with loose cotton wool fixed, without undue pressure, using clear adhesive tape.

DRESSING BROKEN BLISTERS

1 Broken blisters should be covered with sterile dressings (**a**), if available. **2** Add extra padding using cotton wool secured with tape (**b**).

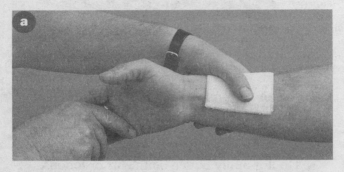

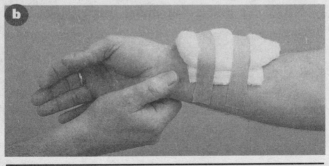

✤ **Do not deliberately cut or prick** a blister. The outer layer of skin forms an ideal dressing over the raw tissue underneath, which is very susceptible to infection.

CHEMICAL BURNS

These are mainly caused by strong acids from car batteries, or alkalis such as caustic soda or strong bleach. Paint strippers and some household cleansers are also corrosive. Take care, in dealing with these situations, not to come into contact with the chemical.

FEATURES

- Stinging sensation of the skin.

- Rapid staining and discoloration.

- Reddening, blistering or peeling.

TREATING A CHEMICAL BURN

1 Immediately and thoroughly wash the affected area under a hose or tap. This will remove surplus material, dilute the chemical and reduce the severity of the burn. If a dry chemical is involved, brush It off with a soft brush first. **2** While washing, remove or cut off any clothing contaminated by the corrosive substance. **3** Cover the burn, if it is inflamed, with a clean cloth or dressing. **4** Get the victim to a hospital.

✣ **Do not waste time** looking for antidotes.

CHEMICAL BURNS OF THE EYE

Alkalis are more dangerous than acids as they penetrate the eye tissues more deeply and are more difficult to remove. The main danger is loss of vision from damage to the outer lens of the eye (the cornea). There is no substitute for immediate, thorough washing.

WASHING AND TREATING THE EYE

1 Hold the victim's head under a tap and let the water run briskly into the eye (**a**). The head should be tilted so that the water runs past the side of the head and not into the undamaged eye. **2** It is essential that the lids should be kept separated during the washing. If the victim cannot do this voluntarily, the lids must be held open (**b**). **3** Maintain the washing for as long as reasonably possible. Ten minutes is not too long for an alkali burn. If both ▶

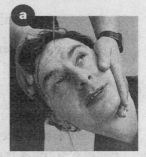

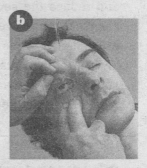

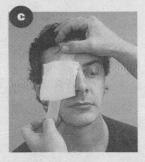

eyes are affected, wash them alternately for 10 seconds each. **4** After irrigation, apply a sterile or clean pad over the closed eye and fix with clear adhesive tape (**c**). **5** Take the victim to a hospital as soon as possible for ophthalmic attention.

◆ **If a tap is not available,** any bland fluid, such as beer, milk or, if all clse fails, urine can be used. Urine is usually sterile and is harmless.

ELECTRICAL BURNS

The first priority is to break the contact between the victim and the electricity supply, without electrocuting yourself.

IN THE EVENT OF
ELECTRIC SHOCK AND BURNS

1 Switch off the current, wrench out the cord or pull out the plug immediately. Switch the electricity off at the box if this is quicker. **2** If necessary, use a broom handle or a wooden chair, while standing on a dry rubber mat, book or folded newspaper, to move the ▶

victim's limb from the point of electrical contact (a). **3** When safe, check the victim's breathing and heartbeat. **4** Attempt artificial ▶

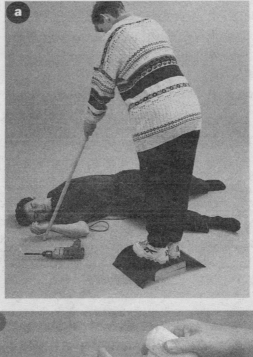

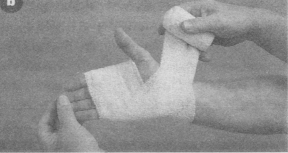

resuscitation and external chest compression (see pp. 7–12), if necessary. **5** Place the victim in the recovery position, if unconscious. **6** Treat the burns, at the points where the electricity entered and left the body, by cooling them with water. **7** Apply a sterile or clean pad and a bandage (**b**).

❖ Never apply water while the victim is still connected to the electricity supply.

HIGH-VOLTAGE ELECTRICITY

Contact with high-voltage electricity, e.g., from an overhead power line, is usually fatal to the victim. You, too, could be killed by "arcing" or jumping electricity, if you are 18 meters (20 yards) or less from the source. Keep other people away and call 911 immediately.

Circulatory Problems

THE CIRCULATORY SYSTEM AND ITS FUNCTION

The brain is the most important organ in the body. The other organs are concerned with its support and maintenance. This is especially true of the heart, which is a muscular pump that keeps blood circulating to the lungs, to pick up oxygen, and to the intestines and liver to pick up fuel, which is mainly in the form of glucose. The essential thing is that blood containing plenty of oxygen and glucose should be continuously supplied to the brain. If this fails, death occurs quickly. So the brain normally has a very good blood supply provided by four large arteries that run up the neck. These branch repeatedly and run all over the surface of the brain sending smaller branches into it. If one of these arteries becomes blocked or there is bleeding from them, a stroke will occur.

The muscles also require oxygen and fuel so that they can perform work by shortening (contracting) to move the body around under the control of the brain. One very important muscle that has to go on contracting continuously, so requiring an especially good oxygen and fuel supply, is the heart muscle. This muscle is supplied with blood by the two coronary arteries (**A**, opposite), which spring from the body's main artery (the aorta) (**B**, opposite) just above the heart, and branch all over the surface of the constantly moving heart. Narrowing of the coronary arteries causes angina (see pp. 96–98); a blockage causes a heart attack (see pp. 100–103).

The heart pumps blood at high pressure into the arteries and receives it back at low pressure by way of the veins. The heart is divided in two (**C**), with right and left sides. The right side (from the person's own point of view) receives blood from the head and body, but not from the lungs, and pumps it to the lungs. Blood from the lungs returns to the left side of the heart which pumps it to the rest of the body. So the blood circulation resembles a "figure-eight." Blood in the arteries of the body (oxgenated blood) is bright red; blood in the veins (deoxygenated blood) is a dark purplish color. The opposite holds for the lung circulation.

THE HEART
a from the head and body
b to the lungs
c to the head and body
d from the lungs

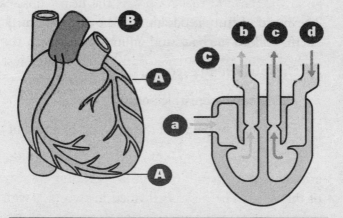

ANGINA

Angina pectoris is a symptom of heart disease, not a disease in itself. It is the pain that originates in the heart muscle when it is trying to perform work without getting enough blood, and hence oxygen and glucose. Blood is supplied to the heart muscle by way of the coronary arteries. If one of the branches of these arteries is severely narrowed by the disease atherosclerosis, it may not be able to carry enough blood to meet the requirements of the heart muscle. Angina is nearly always caused in this way, and nearly always occurs after a fixed amount of exertion or during strong emotional reactions.

<u>FEATURES</u>

- A gripping pain in the center of the chest.

- Spread of the pain down the left or both arms, through to the back and up into the jaw.

- Onset related to exertion.

- There may be breathlessness.

- There may be pallor of the skin and blueness of the lips.

THE AIM OF FIRST AID

The object of the first aider should be to try to reduce, as much as possible, the work of the victim's heart.

♣ **Do not allow** the patient to walk.

IN THE EVENT OF AN ANGINA ATTACK

1 Help the victim to sit down and to assume the most comfortable position. Use rolled-up clothing for padding (**a**). **2** Ask if he has any angina medication (glyceryl-trinitrate) with him. If he does, and it is in pill form, it should ▶

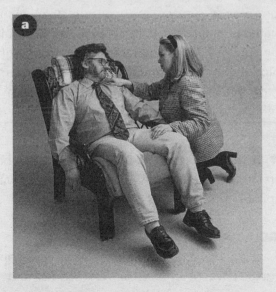

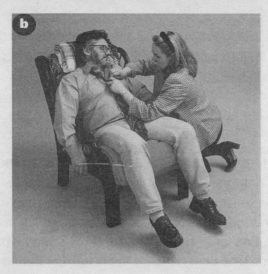

be placed under the tongue (conscious patients only). If it is in spray form, it should be sprayed under the tongue. **3** Loosen tight clothing to ease breathing (**b**). **4** Reassure him. **5** Check that the pain passes within a minute or two of resting.

◆ If the pain persists, this is not angina but a heart attack (see pp. 100–103). Urgent removal to hospital is vital and may save the victim's life.

CARDIAC ARREST

Cardiac arrest means that the heart has stopped beating. This, of course, is very serious and will quickly result in death unless the heart can be restarted.

FEATURES

- The victim collapses and quickly becomes unconscious and motionless.

- There are no breathing movements.

- The pulse cannot be felt anywhere.

- The skin is a gray color.

IN THE EVENT OF CARDIAC ARREST

1 Call for help. **2** Ask someone to call 911. He or she must say that the victim has had a cardiac arrest. **3** Perform two mouth-to-mouth inflations (**a**) (see pp. 7–8). **4** Start external ▶

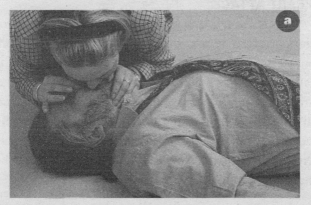

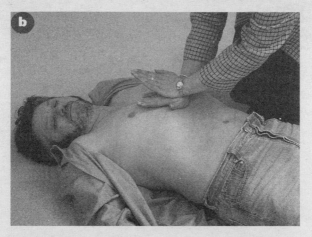

chest compression (**b**) (see pp. 9–12). **5** Give two inflations after every 15 compressions. Continue resuscitation until paramedical help arrives.

HEART ATTACK

This is caused by blockage of a branch of a coronary artery. The part of the heart muscle previously supplied by the blocked branch dies. If the area is large, the victim is unlikely to survive; but if it is small, recovery is possible. In that event, the dead area of muscle is replaced by scar tissue, so the power of the heart is weakened. Some people survive several heart attacks but their hearts may be seriously damaged.

FEATURES

- Sudden onset of crushing central chest pain.

- Pain may spread to arms, back or throat (**a**).

- Conviction that one is dying.

- Faintness and falling.

- Profuse sweating.

- Pale skin.

- Weak, fast pulse. May be irregular. (The average pulse is a steady 60–80 beats per minute.)

- Breathlessness.

- There may be loss of consciousness.

- There may be cardiac arrest (see pp. 98–100).

HEART ATTACK

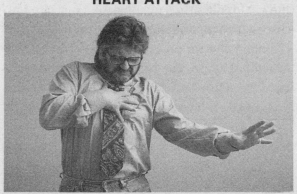

✤ **Do not allow** the victim to move unless it is essential. This will put unnecessary strain on the heart.

✤ **The victim must not be given** anything to eat or drink.

IN THE EVENT OF A HEART ATTACK

1 If the victim is conscious, maneuver him into a half-sitting position. The head, shouders and knees should be supported by cushions (**a**). **2** Reassure the victim and help him to relax. **3** Call for help and ask someone to call 911. He or she must say that the victim has had a heart attack. **4** Loosen tight clothing at the neck, chest and waist (**b**). **5** Check for pulse (see p. 5) and breathing (see p. 2). **6** If the victim becomes unconscious put him into the recovery position (see pp. 16–18) but maintain checks on breathing and pulse. **7** If breathing stops, use mouth-to-mouth resuscitation (see pp. 7–8). **8** If heart stops, start chest compression (see pp. 9–12).

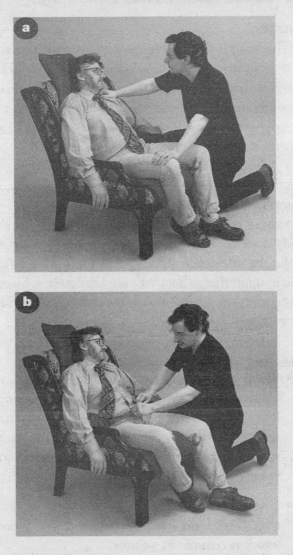

SHOCK

This term is not well understood outside medical circles because the same word is used for "fright." Surgical shock has nothing to do with fright. It is a condition in which either the amount of fluid in the blood vessels is insufficient to fill them or the heart output is not high enough to keep the blood circulating. In either case, the blood pressure drops and the supply of oxygen and fuel to the vital organs, especially the brain, heart and kidneys, is not enough to keep them working properly, if at all. The body does what it can to compensate, by shutting down the arteries to the less vital parts such as the skin and intestines, but there is a limit to this. Shock is very dangerous and, unless corrected, can rapidly prove fatal.

CAUSES

- Blood loss, whether external or internal, e.g., from spinal injury, into the tissues. Serious loss of blood, usually from an artery, may reduce the volume of the blood to the point where there is not enough to fill the blood vessels.

- Loss of fluid by prolonged vomiting or diarrhea. This fluid has to come from the blood, which is reduced in volume.

- Burns. Large quantities of fluid may be lost from the surface or into blisters.

- Infection. Severe blood infection (septicemia) may cause the blood vessels to widen and may lead to leakage of fluid from the blood into the tissues.

- Heart failure. If the heart muscle is weakened it may not be able to keep the blood circulating.

FEATURES

- Pale and cold skin because the skin blood vessels are shut down.

- Rapid pulse because the heart is trying to maintain the circulation.

- Weak pulse because the heart cannot beat strongly.

- The victim feels faint and weak because of the reduced blood supply to the brain and the muscles.

- Severe breathlessness because the blood contains insufficient oxygen.

- Severe thirst because the fluid content of the blood is reduced.

- Possible loss of consciousness because of the reduced blood supply to the brain.

THE AIMS OF FIRST AID

The aims of first aid are to try to prevent the worsening of shock and to make the best use of the limited available circulating blood.

✤ **Do not move** the victim unless it is essential. This could make the shock worse.

✤ **Do not give** the victim anything to eat or drink.

✤ **Do not allow** the victim to smoke.

See box (below) for how to prevent shock from worsening.

PREVENTING SHOCK FROM WORSENING

1 Call 911 or ask someone to telephone for you. **2** The victim should lie down. Keep the head low so that gravity can assist the flow of blood to the brain (**a**). The victim should move as little as possible to keep the heart rate down. **3** Stop any bleeding (see pp. 62–64). **4** Reassure the victim. **5** Loosen tight clothing. **6** Use a folded coat or blanket to raise and support the legs (**b**) so that blood will tend to remain in the central area of the ▶

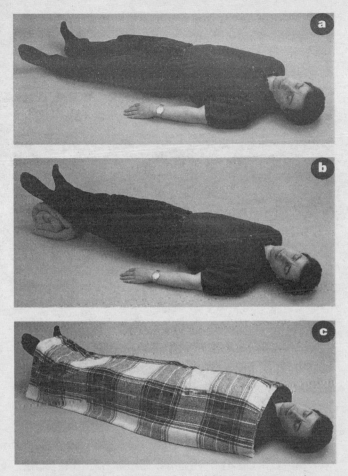

body. **7** Cover the victim with a coat or a single blanket (**c**). **8** Check pulse and breathing at frequent intervals—about every couple of minutes.

✤ **Do not use** a hot water bottle to keep the victim warm. This will attract blood to the skin, diverting it from the major organs.

◆ **If the victim** seems likely to vomit, or if breathing becomes difficult or consciousness is lost, place in the recovery position (**d**) (see pp. 16–18).

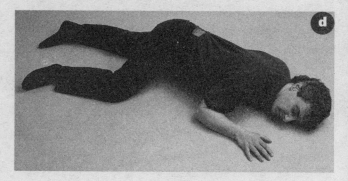

◆ **If the victim's breathing ceases,** begin artificial resuscitation and external chest compression (see pp. 9–12), if necessary.

Crush Injuries

These are the kind of injuries sustained when heavy weights fall on the victims. They occur typically when buildings collapse, mines cave in or during the course of serious industrial accidents or earthquakes. In addition to the usual injuries, such as fractures and wounds, crush injuries have special features that affect first aid management. Crushed muscle releases muscle hemoglobin into the blood and this can clog up the kidneys, preventing them from working. Considerable quantities of blood can be lost into crushed muscle.

FEATURES

- Presence of a heavy weight across a muscular part.

- Severe swelling, bruising and blistering around crushed area.

- No pulse beyond crushed area.

- Limb cold and pale beyond point of crushing.

- Probable shock (see pp. 104–108).

- Indications of fractures (see pp. 121–122).

THE IMPORTANCE OF TIME

First aid depends on how long the crushing force has been present.

LESS THAN ONE HOUR

1 Remove the crushing weight as quickly as possible (**a**). **2** Get help quickly if you are alone. **3** Call 911. **4** Check the injuries. **5** Check breathing (see p. 2) and pulse (**b**) (see p. 5).

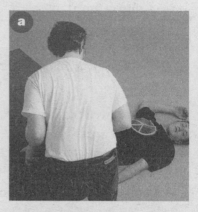

6 Control any external bleeding (see pp. 62–64). **7** Treat as for shock (see pp. 104–108). **8** If the victim becomes unconscious place him in the recovery position (see pp. 16–18).

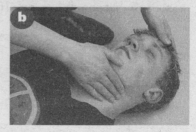

9 Make a note of how long the crushing force persisted and of the time of release. Inform the medical authorities.

✤ **Do not allow** the victim to move.

MORE THAN ONE HOUR

1 Leave the weight in place and explain why to the victim. **2** Call the emergency services and explain the nature of the problem. **3** Reassure the victim.

✣ **After 1 hour, removing the weight** may do more harm than good.

Dislocations

Dislocations occur at joints when the bones forming the joints are forced into an abnormal relationship. The force may also cause a fracture (see pp. 120–123). Dislocations involve either tearing of the soft tissues, such as ligaments and joint capsules, or occur because they are abnormally lax. Any joint can suffer a dislocation but some joints are more dependent on support from soft tissues than others and are, consequently, more likely to suffer dislocation. The most commonly dislocated joint is the shoulder. Dislocations are also fairly common in the jaw and the thumb.

FEATURES
• Abnormal shape and appearance of the joint.

- Loss of use of the joint.

- Swelling and bruising around the joint.

- Usually severe pain, unless the dislocation has occurred many times before.

DISLOCATED SHOULDER

The head of the upper arm bone (humerus) sits in a very shallow hollow in the side of the shoulder blade (a) and is easily displaced downwards and inwards (b). Dislocation usually results from a fall on the outstretched hand. The capsule of the joint tears and the head of the bone slips though the gap.

FEATURES

- The arm appears too long and the profile of the shoulder appears abnormal with a sharp angle (b).

- The casualty may prefer to support the arm on the dislocated side with the other hand.

✤ **Do not attempt to move** or "click" the bones back into position. This could damage the surrounding nerves and tissue or, if one is present, make the fracture worse.

IN THE EVENT OF DISLOCATION

1 Support the injured shoulder in the most comfortable position. **2** Maintain it in this position with a pillow or cushion (**c**), sling or bandages (see pp. 193–196). **3** Arrange for transport to a hospital.

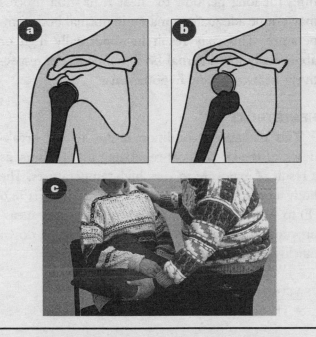

♣ **Avoid giving food or drink,** as a general anaesthetic may be needed.

Extremes of Body Temperature

The body has excellent temperature regulating mechanisms and can normally be relied on to keep internal temperature within narrow limits. If, however, the body is exposed to high or low temperatures for long periods, the heat regulation process may not be adequate to maintain normal body temperature. This may result in abnormally high or abnormally low internal body temperature: respectively, heatstroke and hypothermia.

HEATSTROKE

This dangerous condition is due to the breakdown of the body's heat-regulating mechanisms, as a result of exposure to very high temperatures. The body temperature rises from the normal 37 °C (98.6 °F) to 41 °C (105.8 °F) or higher. Emergency measures are necessary to get the temperature down quickly if life is to be saved.

FEATURES

- The victim may become unconscious.

- The victim is restless and dizzy.

- The victim complains of feeling hot and having a headache.

- The skin is hot and dry.

- The pulse is strong and fast.

- The victim may become confused.

- Coma may result.

MANAGEMENT OF HEATSTROKE

1 Summon medical help and explain what is happening. **2** Place the victim in a half-lying, half-sitting position. **3** Remove all the victim's clothing. **4** Wrap him in a cold wet sheet. **5** Keep the sheet wet with cold water. **6** Fan the sheet so that evaporation cools the victim more effectively. **7** Stop when the skin feels cool or the temperature falls to 38 °C (100.4 °F). **8** Watch out for a second rise in body temperature. Repeat steps 4 to 6, if necessary.

◆ **If the victim is unconscious,** cool him in the recovery position (see pp. 16–18). Check breathing and pulse (see pp. 2 and 5).

HYPOTHERMIA

This condition arises where the body's temperature drops below the normal level of 37 °C (98.6 °F). If, for example, heat is constantly carried away by cold winds, the body's heat-production process (shivering) may cease to function adequately. Elderly and frail people, especially if thin, tired and hungry, are most liable to hypothermia, particularly in inadequately heated or unheated houses.

FEATURES

- There is early shivering, which may pass off.

- The skin is cold and dry.

- The pulse is slow.

- The victim's rate of breathing is slow.

- The measured body temperature is 35 °C (95 °F) or less.

- There is drowsiness which may progress to coma.

- There may be cardiac arrest (see pp. 98–100).

AIMS OF FIRST AID

The aim is to warm the body gradually but with minimum delay. Never assume that a hypothermic victim has died unless this is obvious. Hypothermia protects the brain against lack of oxygen and a person can survive a longer than usual period of cardiac arrest.

MANAGEMENT OF HYPOTHERMIA: OUTDOORS

1 Send for medical help. **2** Get the victim into a sheltered place or indoors as soon as possible. **3** Use a sleeping bag, or other form of insulation, to cover the victim. **4** Share your own body heat with the victim under a common cover. **5** Check for breathing (see p. 2). **6** Check for pulse (see p. 5). **7** Give hot drinks and food, if available.

MANAGEMENT OF HYPOTHERMIA: INDOORS

1 Send for medical help. **2** If the victim is conscious and uninjured, put him in a warmed bed. Make sure the head (but not the face) is covered, too. **3** Give hot drinks and food.

◆ **If the victim is unconscious,** resuscitate, if necessary, by mouth-to-mouth resuscitation and chest compression.

✣ **Do not rub** the victim's limbs or encourage vigorous movement.

✤ **Do not allow** the victim to drink any alcohol. This causes heat loss.

✤ **Do not immerse** the victim in a hot bath or use hot water bottles. This will divert blood from the major organs to the superficial vessels of the skin.

FROSTBITE

Frostbite is most dangerous when it causes the freezing of blood vessels, which can then cut off the blood supply to the affected area and may result in gangrene.

Extremities, such as the nose tip, the fingers and the toes, are most at risk. When frostbitten they initially become cold, hard and white, and then red and swollen.

MANAGEMENT OF FROSTBITE

1 Get the affected person under shelter.
2 Put the frozen parts into water at 40 °C (104 °F). **3** Get medical attention.

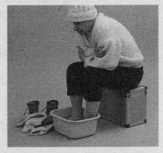

✤ **Avoid movement:** keep the frozen parts still in the water and do not massage them.

HEAT EXHAUSTION

Heat exhaustion is caused by excessive loss of fluid and salt from the body. The following features are displayed.

FEATURES

- Pale, clammy skin.
- Faintness.
- Dizziness.
- Headaches.
- Nausea.
- Muscle cramps.
- Rapid pulse.
- Fast, shallow breathing.

TREATING HEAT EXHAUSTION

1 The victim should lie down in a cool place.
2 Elevate the legs (a). **3** The victim should, ▶

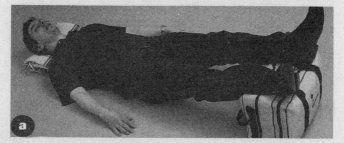

slowly but continuously, drink weak salt
water (**b**) (at a ratio of
half a level teaspoon
of salt per quart of
water) until his condi-
tion improves. **4** Call
a doctor.

FALLING UNCONSCIOUS

If the victim falls unconscious, put them into the
recovery position (see pp. 16–18) and call 911.

Fractures

CAUSES AND SITES OF FRACTURE

Any bone in the body can be fractured by direct
violence, by bending or twisting, by force transmitted along a bone, by excessive stress from the muscle pull or by disease that weakens bone. Old bones
break more easily and more cleanly than young
bones, which often suffer incomplete (greenstick)
fractures.

Some fractures are more common than others.
The sites of the most common fractures are shown
opposite.

SITES OF FRACTURE

a skull
b collarbone
c ribs
d elbow
e pelvis
f neck of the thigh
   bone
g shaft of thigh
   bone
h ankle
i nose, jaw and
   cheekbone
j breastbone
k upper arm
l spine
m lower arm bones
n wrist
o toes and fingers
p kneecap
q lower leg bones

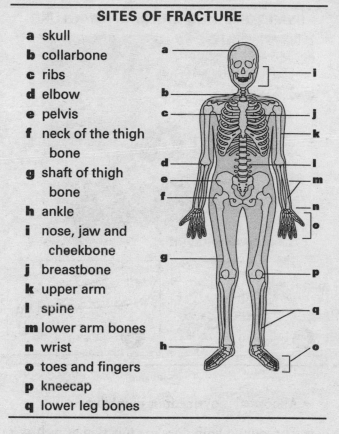

SYMPTOMS AND SIGNS OF FRACTURE

- Pain and tenderness to touch (**a**).

- Swelling, bruising (**b**) and deformity (**c**), such as
  irregularity in the line of the bone or shortening
  of the affected limb.

SYMPTOMS AND SIGNS OF FRACTURE

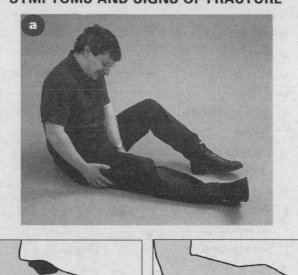

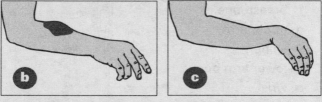

- Abnormal movement or instability.

- The injured limb does not function as well as it did, if at all.

- A grating sensation on attempts at movement (crepitus).

- There may be features of shock (see p. 105).

✤ **Do not move** a victim with a fracture unless it is absolutely essential.

✤ **No attempt** should ever be made to test for crepitus. This may cause further injury.

IMMOBILIZATION AND MANAGEMENT OF FRACTURES

GENERAL PRINCIPLES

- Avoid all unnecessary movements at the fracture site.

- With leg fractures, move the victim only if he or she is in a dangerous situation.

- Check the pulse beyond the fracture site. If you think there is no pulse treat the matter as very urgent.

- Call 911 and explain in detail what has happened.

- Remember that paramedic ambulance personnel are equipped with excellent splints for fractures and that you might delay matters by applying makeshift splints.

- You can, however, make a person with an arm or hand or collar bone fracture much more comfortable by applying padding and a supporting sling.

- Open fractures call for special attention (see below).

- Neck or spinal fractures are particularly dangerous and must be handled with great care (see pp. 127 and 130).

- If you must apply emergency splints, remember that a fracture will not be immobilized unless the splints prevent movement in the joint above and the joint below the fracture.

- Always pad the fracture site carefully and avoid undue pressure on it unless this is necessary to control severe bleeding.

- A leg fracture can be immobilized by strapping both legs together after padding well.

- Rib fractures may be associated with a sucking wound through which air is passing. If so the wound must be sealed off immediately and effectively. You can save a life by doing this. Use your hand while calling for a suitable pad, which must be fixed firmly in place.

OPEN FRACTURES
FEATURES

- There is always a wound near the fracture site.

- Protruding bone ends might be visible.

WHERE THE BONE IS NOT PROTRUDING
1 Call 911. **2** If there is much bleeding, apply pressure if possible (**a**). **3** Squeeze the edges

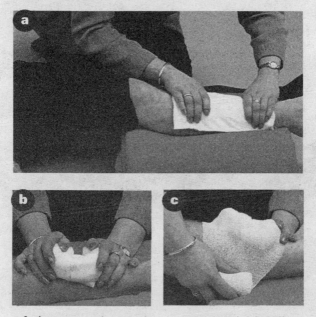

of the wound together, to control bleeding (see pp. 62–64). **4** Cover with a pad (**a**) of clean material such as a folded handkerchief. Use sterile gauze, if available (**b**). **5** Secure the covering with a pad and a firm bandage (**c**) (see pp. 174–176). **6** Immobilize the injured part (see pp. 193–196) and get the victim to a hospital.

✤ **Do not tie** the bandage too tight as this might impair circulation.

✤ **While performing this procedure,** avoid moving the fracture by supporting the part fully with your hand.

WHERE THE BONE PROTRUDES

1 Place sterile gauze, if available, or a piece of clean cloth over the wound (**a**). **2** Place a ring ▶

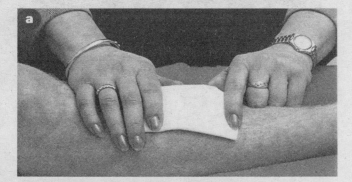

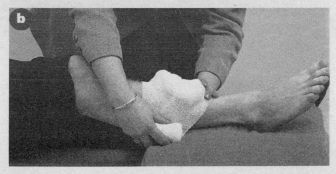

of cotton wool around the open wound, over the gauze. It must be higher than the protruding bone. **3** Fix this in place with a secure, diagonally-placed bandage (**b**) (see pp. 187–188). **4** Immobilize the part. **5** Arrange for the victim's transport to a hospital.

❖ **Be careful to avoid** movement at the fracture site at all times. Give the injured part full support with your hands.

NECK FRACTURES
The neck and spine
  a neck
  b spine

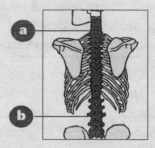

FEATURES

• The victim may have a stiff neck.

• They may be unable to move arms or legs.

• There may be tingling or loss of sensation below the level of the fracture.

IMMOBILIZATION AND MANAGEMENT

1 Call 911 immediately. **2** Leave victim flat on the back. **3** Reassure the victim. **4** Squat above and behind the victim's head and keep the head straight with

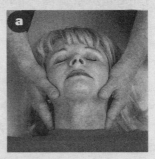

your hands over the ears (**a**). **5** A firm (cervical) collar around the neck, made from rolled-up newspaper can help, but you must continue to hold the head straight.

✤ **Do not move** the victim unless essential to ensure his or her safety (see pp. 30–31). Improper movement can lead to permanent total paralysis or death.

✤ **Do not remove** a crash helmet unless the airway is blocked, or if there is no breathing or no pulse. For crash helmet removal, see pp. 55–57.

MAKING AND APPLYING
A CERVICAL COLLAR

Two first aiders will be required. The collar can be applied either for a patient sitting or lying down. **1** Roll a newspaper in cloth (**b**). ▶

2 Place the center of the collar under the chin and wrap it around the neck (**c**). **3** Secure it with a scarf knotted at the front (**d**).
4 Check the breathing.

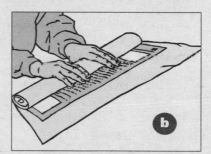

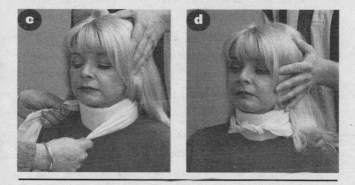

❖ **The head should be held** absolutely still during and after the application of the collar.

❖ **Do not wrap** the collar around the neck too tightly.

◆ **If there is no suitable paper available,** the head should be held until professional help arrives.

SPINE FRACTURES

<u>FEATURES</u>

- There may be severe back pain.

- There may be loss of use of legs and arms.

- There may be tingling or loss of sensation below the fracture.

IMMOBILIZATION AND MANAGEMENT

Two first aiders will be required. **1** Tell the victim to try not to move. **2** Check breathing (see p. 2) and circulation (see p. 5). **3** Call 911 immediately. **4** One person should squat above and behind the victim's head, holding it with the hands over the victim's ears (**a**). The head should be kept straight. **5** Support the victim's trunk with rolled-up clothes on either side (**b**). **6** Put soft padding between the legs and bind them together at hips, thighs and ankles (**c**). **7** If vomiting is imminent, turn ▶

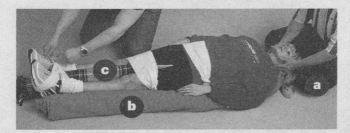

the victim into the spinal recovery position (below). **8** Make sure that the airway remains clear. **9** Transport the victim to a hospital, lying down.

✤ **Do not move** the victim unless it is essential to ensure safety (see pp. 30–31 and 47–49). Improper movement can lead to permanent total paralysis or death.

SPINAL RECOVERY POSITION

This must be adopted only if the victim is unconscious. **1** Six people are required. One ensures that the head, neck and body always remain in line, to avoid further injury. This person gives orders to the others (**a**). **2** Three ▶

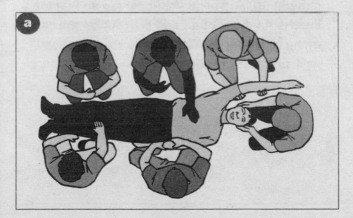

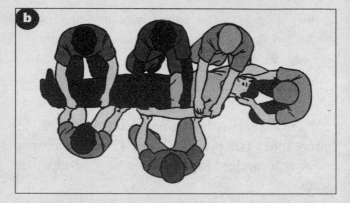

people kneel on one side, two on the other. **3** Apply a neck collar (see pp. 128–129). **4** The three helpers must carefully roll the victim on to the side with the raised arm, avoiding twisting the spine, while the two on the other side carefully lift (**b**). **5** Move the victim's lower arm under the head to help keep the neck straight (**c**), and bend the upper leg so that the knee is on the ground and the foot on the calf of the other leg (**d**). Continue to keep the head, neck and body in alignment.

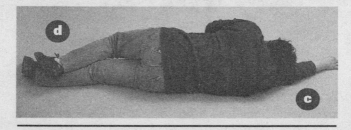

Muscle Injuries

GENERAL MUSCLE INJURIES

The body contains hundreds of muscles and any of them can be injured. In practice, injuries most commonly affect the muscles of the limbs and the back. Muscles may be bruised, stretched, torn, lacerated or pulled off their attachment to bone. The severity of the injury can usually be judged by the degree of disablement. Severe muscle injuries are often associated with fractures and should be checked by a doctor.

FEATURES

- Pain and tenderness when the injured part is pressed.

- Bruising, swelling and stiffness.

- Cramps may occur.

- Loss of the affected muscle's ability to function.

MANAGEMENT OF MUSCLE INJURIES

1 Sit or lay the injured person down. **2** Put the injured part in the most comfortable position. If the affected part is a limb, elevate it. **3** Apply a cold pack (ice-pack or a pack of frozen ▶

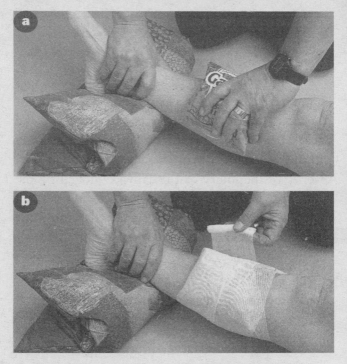

food, such as peas) (**a**), bandage it in place and leave for half an hour. This will limit internal bleeding and bruising. **4** Firmly compress the injured part with a thick layer of cotton wool bound on with a bandage (**b**). This will help to reduce swelling.

4

Minor Injuries
and Conditions

Many of the conditions dealt with in this section of the book are not serious enough to warrant medical attention. Some of them, however, can be potentially dangerous, and these always require medical attention. Minor injuries are far more common than serious injuries, and in most cases require only simple remedies. As a rule, full recovery is to be expected. If the problem persists, however, it is advisable to consult a doctor.

Aches and Pains

BACKACHE

There are many causes of backache, some serious, some not (for serious injuries see pp. 130–132). In most cases back pain does not imply that anything serious has happened, but consult a doctor if any of the following features occur.

FEATURES

- Severe pain.

- Persistent pain.

- Numbness or weakness in a leg.

- Problems with bladder and/or bowel control.

RELIEVING BACKACHE

1 Apply local heat to the back from a hot-water bottle or heat lamp. **2** Use of pain relieving drugs, such as aspirin, acetamino-phen or ibuprofen for short periods, should only be administered by the patient.

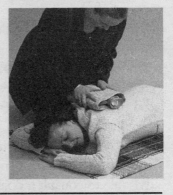

◆ **If the pain does not settle** in a day or two, consult a doctor.

HEADACHE

The great majority of headaches are caused by muscle tension responding in turn to psychological tension. There are also other, less frequent, causes of headaches.

CAUSES
- Excessive alcohol consumption.
- Hunger.
- Tiredness.
- Oppressive weather.
- Migraine.
- Allergies.

Only a very small proportion of headaches indicate a serious condition, such as a brain tumor, high blood pressure or an aneurysm (where artery swelling occurs). Visual difficulties seldom cause headaches.

RELIEVING HEADACHES

1 The victim should relax.
2 Use pain relievers.
3 Apply a cold compress or covered hot-water bottle to the forehead.

HEADACHES OCCURRING FOR NO OBVIOUS REASON

Such headaches should be reported and investigated. This is particularly important in the case of headaches associated with other symptoms, such as weakness or loss of sensation, or loss of parts of the field of vision.

EARACHE

This is particularly common in children, in whom it is usually due to infection in the middle ear (**a**; see below) or in the passage (**b**; see below) leading to the ear drum (**c**; see below). Other cases may be due to a small boil in the ear passage.

CROSS-SECTION OF THE EAR

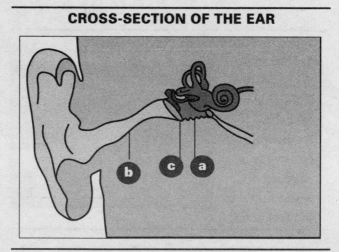

Consult a doctor if any of the following features are present.

FEATURES
- Fever.
- Deafness.
- Discharge from the ear.

RELIEVING EARACHE

1 Self-help is limited to giving pain relieving drugs. **2** Check the victim's temperature and consult a doctor if a fever is developing.

◆ **If the pain persists** for more than a day, consult a doctor.

✤ **Avoid giving aspirin to children** under 12 due to Reye's Syndrome. Use acetaminophen or ibuprofen in suitable dosage.

MENSTRUAL PAIN

Painful periods are very common and do not usually imply anything very serious.

RELIEVING MENSTRUAL PAIN

1 Use pain relievers such as ibuprofen, aspirin or acetaminophen. **2** When the pain is ▶

particularly severe, take a hot bath and then relax for a time in bed, preferably with a hot-water bottle.

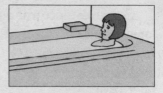

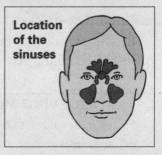

◆ **If the pain is very severe and persistent,** consult a doctor—it may be due to serious disorders, such as pelvic infection or hormone imbalance, or to some other gynecological problem.

THE COMBINED ORAL CONTRACEPTIVE PILL

In many cases, the contraceptive pill is an effective way of treating very severe menstrual pains. Because it prevents egg production (ovulation), cycles usually bring less or no pain.

SINUS PAIN

Acute sinusitis commonly follows a cold and causes pain—often throbbing—above, below or

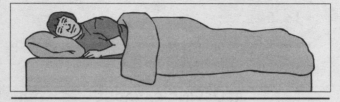

Location of the sinuses

between the eyes. The pain may be associated with fever, in which case medical attention is advised.

METHODS OF RELIEVING SINUS PAIN

1 Use decongestant tablets or a decongestant nasal spray. It is often helpful to inhale the vapor from hot water in a bowl, with a towel over the head. **2** Tincture of benzoin inhalations are also commonly used for sinusitis. They are available without prescription.

TOOTHACHE

Toothache is pain occurring in the jaws or teeth, which may be continuous, intermittent or throbbing. There are several different causes of toothache.

CAUSES

- Dental decay, with infection of the tooth pulp (a).

- Exposure of sensitive dentine at the necks of the teeth.

- Deep, unlined fillings.

- Tooth fractures.

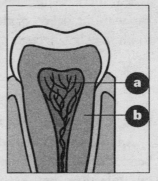

METHODS OF RELIEVING TOOTHACHE

There are several ways to relieve toothache.

1 If sharp toothache occurs on contact with acids, fruits or ice cream, it can probably be relieved by using a toothpaste that seals the tubules in the dentine (**b**).

2 The affected tooth can be dabbed with oil of cloves (**c**). 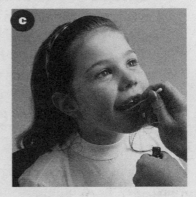 **3** The victim can place a covered hot-water bottle against the painful side of the face.

4 Pain relievers may be taken.

◆ **If there is still pain** the victim should see a dentist without delay as the pulp (**a**) of the affected tooth may be infected.

Bites and Stings

DOG, CAT AND HUMAN BITES

Animal and human mouths contain large numbers of organisms, some capable of producing serious infections and even potentially fatal diseases, such as rabies. Bites that penetrate the skin must, therefore, always be taken seriously.

MANAGEMENT OF BITES

1 Immediately wash the bite well with plenty of soap and water. **2** Allow the bite to bleed naturally, in order to carry away germs. **3** Apply gauze soaked in hydrogen peroxide, in order to reduce the risk of infection. **4** Report the bite to a doctor, as tetanus immunization and antibiotics may be required. **5** If rabies is suspected, the victim must be taken to a hospital.

VERIFICATION OF RABIES

In order to verify or exclude a rabies infection, the suspect animal must prove its vaccinations are current, or if it is feral, undergo medical examination. Attempt to isolate the animal only if it is possible to do so safely. If a suspect animal escapes, inform the police at once.

SNAKEBITES

Snakebites are rare in the United States and are seldom serious, hardly ever causing death. Pit vipers and coral snakes are the most common poisonous species in the United States, with pit viper bites accounting for 98 percent of all poisonous snake bites each year. In other parts of the world, other types of snakes, such as cobras, kraits, and mambas, are common and cause many deaths.

The medical authorities in areas of high prevalence of poisonous snakes hold stocks of antivenom and are experienced in the management of snakebites.

<u>FEATURES</u>

- There is pain and swelling around the bite.

- One or two puncture wounds are evident.

- The victim's vision may deteriorate.

- There is nausea and there may be vomiting.

- There may be breathing difficulty.

MANAGEMENT OF SNAKEBITES

1 The victim must be made to rest (**a**) in order to slow the heart down, thereby reducing ▶

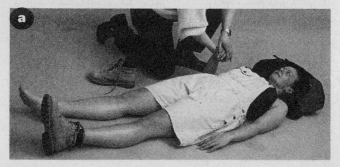

poison absorption. **2** Clean the wound by wiping away from the bite (**b**), to remove any venom that may be around the wound. **3** Bandage the wound firmly (**c**). **4** Get the victim to a hospital or to a doctor as quickly as possible.

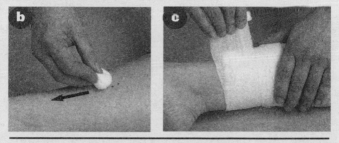

✤ Do not let the victim move.
✤ Do not elevate the injured limb.
✤ Do not cut into or cauterize the bite.

INSECT BITES

These are not really bites but are usually the effect of a small quantity of material in the insect's saliva, which is injected into the skin via the insect's proboscis. The material causes an allergic reaction—taking the form of redness, swelling and irritation—which usually settles in a day or two. Some reactions are caused by insect feces scratched into the skin. Occasionally, severe reactions occur which may be life-threatening, especially if swelling occurs in the voice-box (larynx).

TREATING INSECT BITES

1 Wash the skin area thoroughly with soap and water. **2** All severe local or general reactions should receive medical treatment urgently.

STINGS

Stings by bees, wasps, hornets, jellyfish, etc., involve the injection of highly irritating venom, which, while causing severe local pain, redness and swelling, is usually fairly harmless. Very large numbers of simultaneous stings, however, may be dangerous. Also dangerous are general allergic reactions to a single sting in a person who has become sensitized by a previous sting.

TREATING STINGS

1 Sting sacs left protruding from the skin must be carefully scraped off with a blunt knife blade **(a)** or a fingernail. **2** Wash the affected area ▸

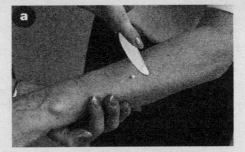

with soap and water (**b**) and apply an ice cube
(**c**). **3** Administer pain relievers to the victim.

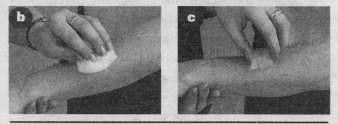

✣ **Avoid using tweezers** to remove the sting, as
this will squeeze the venom into the skin.

STINGS IN THE MOUTH OR THROAT
In this instance, the victim must be taken to a
doctor or hospital casualty department immediately.
Such stings may cause fatal swelling of the voice-
box with obstruction of the airway.

GENERAL ALLERGIC REACTIONS
Any general allergic reactions require immediate
medical attention.

IF A PERSON COLLAPSES AFTER A STING
1 Check the breathing (see p. 2). **2** Check the
pulse (see p. 5). **3** Perform mouth-to-mouth
artificial resuscitation (see pp. 7–8) and chest
compression (see pp. 9–12), if necessary.

Black Eye

The skin of the eyelids is very thin and covers many large veins. A black eye (**a**) results from a blow or fall that damages these veins and releases blood into the surrounding tissues, thereby darkening the area.

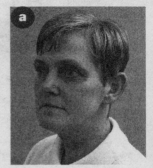

Once the blood has been released there is nothing to be done but to wait for it to be absorbed. This will take two to three weeks (depending on the severity of bruising), during which time the skin around the eye will pass through a series of varied colors.

TREATING A BLACK EYE

1 Place an ice pack (such as a pack of frozen peas) on the eye area (**b**) immediately after the injury has been sustained, in order to minimize its prominence. **2** Check the vision in the affected eye as soon ▸

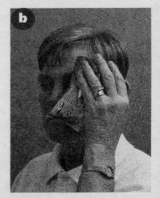

as possible. **3** If vision
seems impaired, then
the victim's eyelids
should be pulled
slightly open with fin-
gers (**c**) and the vision
compared with that of
the other eye. **4** The
eyes should be moved

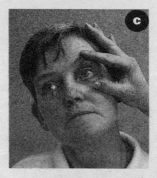

from side to side and up and down to check
for double vision.

PROBLEMS WITH VISION

Consult a doctor immediately if there is any
visual problem of any kind.

Bleeding

Minor bleeding seldom presents any serious problems unless the person concerned is suffering from a
bleeding disorder, such as hemophilia.

Minor bleeding always results from damage to
small blood vessels, such as venules (small veins) or
capillaries. Pulsating spurts of bright red blood from
an artery, however small, can never be considered
minor and will always require medical attention (see
pp. 20–21 and 62–64).

The principle behind the various methods of

bleeding control remains the same in all cases: apply pressure at once and sustain it. Different forms of bleeding, however, call for the pressure to be applied in different ways.

MINOR WOUNDS, CUTS AND GRAZES

The surface of the skin (**a**) offers excellent protection against infection, but once the surface is breached, whether by a cut (**b**) or an abrasion (see p. 58 for types of minor wound), infection of the sterile underlying tissues (**c**) is likely.

SECTION THROUGH THE SKIN WITH CUT

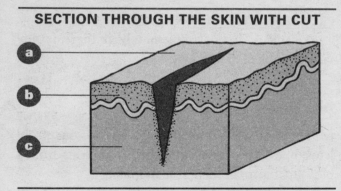

In most cases, the body's defense mechanisms can cope with any such infection, and the wound heals after a short period of inflammation. From time to time, however, minor cuts are contaminated with very dangerous (virulent) organisms, and serious infections, such as blood poisoning, may result.

TREATING A MINOR WOUND

1 Wash the wound and the surrounding skin thoroughly with soap and water (**a**) as soon as a minor wound, cut or graze is oustained.

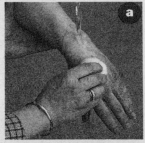

2 Remove any foreign material and dirt from the wound. **3** Wash hands, and then shake them dry. **4** Swab the skin around the wound with an antiseptic solution (**b**) (checking the instructions on the bottle for correct usage).

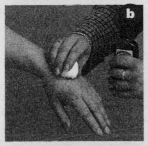

5 Apply a sterile dressing or Band-Aid-type bandage (**c**) after the wound has been thoroughly cleaned. Leave the dressing in place until the wound has

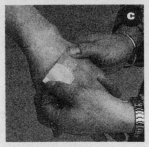

healed. Disturb it only if it comes loose or becomes very dirty.

✤ **Do not touch the wound,** even with a clean towel.

✤ **Avoid touching the surface of the dressing** that comes in contact with the wound.

✤ **Do not use a towel for drying hands** unless it is newly laundered. Used towels carry germs which can contaminate the wound.

◆ **If the wound is still not comfortable** after the first day, and is accompanied by increasing pain, heat, swelling or throbbing, then a doctor must be consulted.

HEALING TIME

Minor wounds which are properly treated will usually heal in about a week.

DEEP WOUNDS

Deep wounds should always be reported, however small. Even a very small deep wound is potentially dangerous, especially if the object causing the wound was contaminated. Cultivated soil, for example, often contains dangerous organisms, and a puncture wound sustained while gardening can have grave consequences.

NOSEBLEEDS

The nose contains many blood vessels, which lie close to the inner surface of the nose lining. These vessels bleed readily if they are injured by external force, or if the nose is blown too hard or over-enthusiastically explored! Nosebleeds are seldom serious.

STOPPING A NOSEBLEED

1 Pinch the nostrils in the area immediately below the nasal bones firmly with the thumb and forefinger (**a**) as soon as a nosebleed is recognized. **2** The victim should sit down with head forward over a washbowl (**b**). **3** The pressure on the bleeding vessels must be maintained for at least ten minutes, and the victim must not raise the head. **4** Release the pressure gradu- ally. **5** With the head still forward, wipe carefully around the ▶

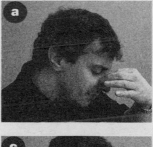

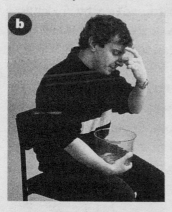

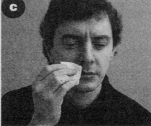

mouth and nose with a clean dressing or swab
which has been soaked in lukewarm water (**c**).

♣ **The victim must avoid blowing the nose** for
at least four hours after the bleeding has stopped, if
this is at all possible.

◆ **If the bleeding continues,** steps 1 to 5 should
be repeated.

◆ **If the bleeding still continues,** then the victim
must be taken to a hospital emergency room. The
victim must still hold the nose.

GUM AND TOOTH SOCKET BLEEDING

BLEEDING FROM THE GUMS

This usually occurs while tooth-brushing; it
nearly always implies gum disease, such as gingivi-
tis, and suggests that there has been neglect of tooth
hygiene. This is a matter for advice by a dentist.
Gum bleeding from injury is seldom persistent and
will usually stop on application of pressure.

BLEEDING FROM A TOOTH SOCKET

This occasionally follows a tooth extraction or
the accidental loss of a tooth. It can also occur after
a fracture of the jaw has been incurred. The first two
cases require the following approach.

STOPPING TOOTH SOCKET BLEEDING

1 Apply pressure to the socket by means of a pad of some kind. Use a small, clean handkerchief, or other piece of clean cloth, rolled into a small cylinder that will fit between the teeth on either side of the gap, while protruding well above the level of the teeth margins (**a**). **2** Bite firmly on the cloth so as to force it against the socket (**b**). Maintain the pressure for at least 10 minutes. **3** Release the bite pressure gradually.

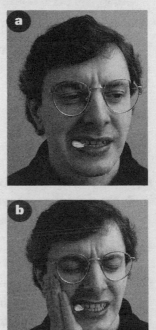

◆ **If the tooth socket continues to bleed,** it may be necessary to maintain the pressure for longer than this or to repeat the procedure.

✤ **Avoid pulling out any blood clot** that has formed by removing the cloth carefully.

◆ **If the blood clot still comes out,** try lubricating the cloth with a little sterile vaseline before putting it back in.

◆ **If this method still fails to stop the bleeding,** seek help from a dentist or a hospital emergency room.

Burns

See pp. 80–93 for management of major burns.

MINOR BURNS AND SCALDS

✤ **Do not interfere with the blister** by pricking it or removing any loose skin.

TREATING MINOR BURNS AND SCALDS

1 All burns, however minor, should be treated by immediate cooling to minimize tissue damage. Get the injured part under a gushing cold tap (**a**) as quickly as possible, and keep it ◗

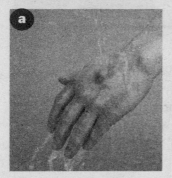
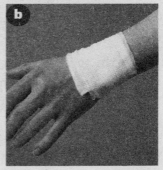

there until thoroughly cooled. **2** Dress the burn with clean, non-fluffy material (**b**) (see pp. 88 and 175–176) which is preferably sterile.

SUNBURN

Sunburn is caused by excessive exposure to the sun's rays. Sunlight contains ultraviolet rays which destroy cells in the outer layer of the skin and damage the small blood vessels which lie beneath the skin. Sunburn can vary from mild burning to severe blistering. It has two effects.

EFFECTS

- Immediate discomfort and inconvenience.

- Long-term increase in the risk of skin wrinkling and skin cancer.

RELIEVING SUNBURN

1 Get out of the sun. **2** Cool the skin under a cold shower. **3** Avoid pressure on the burnt skin. **4** In cases of mild sunburn apply witch hazel, natural ▶

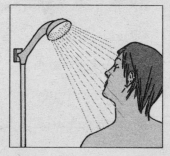

yogurt, calamine lotion or a proprietary lotion or cream. **5** Try to preserve blisters in more serious cases. **6** Use pain relievers. **7** Seek medical advice if burning is severe.

Fainting

Fainting is a brief loss of consciousness due to a temporary shortage of blood to the brain. This usually occurs because of widening of the blood vessels of the body, so that the blood volume is inadequate to maintain the pressure in the uppermost parts. Occasionally, a faint is caused by an undue slowing of the heart. More usual causes, however, are listed below.

CAUSES

- Stuffy or overheated environments.

- Prolonged standing.

- Fear or severe distress.

- Pain.

- Prolonged coughing.

- Straining during defecation.

A victim will usually display some of the following features.

FEATURES
- Pallor.
- Sweating.
- Dizziness.
- Dimming of vision.
- Ringing in the ears.
- Loss of consciousness.
- Falling down.

MANAGEMENT OF FAINTING
1 The victim should lie down. **2** Raise the legs high. **3** Loosen tight clothing.

❖ Do not raise the victim to an upright position.
❖ If the airway becomes noisy, place patient in the recovery position.

Fevers

A fever is defined as a rise in body temperature above the normal 37 °C (98.6 °F). Fevers have a variety of causes.

CAUSES

- The most common cause is bacterial or viral infection.

- Overactive thyroid gland.

- Excessive loss of body fluid.

- Excessive heat to the head.

- Heart attack.

- Lymphoma tumor.

TREATING FEVERS

1 Remove all clothes. **2** Sponge down repeatedly with cool-to-tepid water. **3** If feasible, put the fevered person in a cool-to-tepid bath. **4** Give aspirin, unless otherwise advised. **5** All fevers should be reported to a doctor.

✤ **Very high fever must not be allowed to persist:** it may result in brain damage.

✤ **Never give aspirin to a fevered child** under 12 years of age: it may provoke Reye's syndrome—a serious liver and brain disorder.

Foreign Bodies

Children commonly put small foreign bodies—such as beads, stones, ball bearings, marbles, peas or beans—in their ears and noses. Also, objects, such as fish hooks or splinters, may acidentally become lodged in parts of the body, which need removal. Organic foreign bodies can absorb moisture and swell, so that removal becomes difficult.

FOREIGN BODIES IN THE EAR

Insects sometimes crawl or fly into the ear passage. They cannot get beyond the eardrum and remain in the outer passage, sometimes stuck to soft wax, until removed. A live insect will sometimes cause loud noises by striking the eardrum. This is harmless.

REMOVING INSECTS FROM THE EAR

If it is certain that there is an insect in the ear passage, it might be floated out by gently ▶

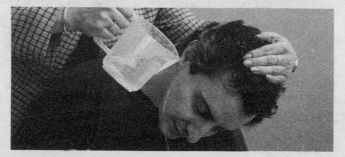

pouring lukewarm water into the ear from a small pitcher.

◆ **If the insect remains in the ear,** then a doctor will have to be consulted.

✢ **Do not try to remove solid foreign bodies:** attempts to do so will invariably push them further into the ear passage. Get the victim to a doctor.

FOREIGN BODIES IN THE EYE

Small foreign bodies can frequently obstruct the eye area. There are several places where they may be found.

AREAS OF THE EYE LIKELY TO BE AFFECTED

• The outside of the eye.

• Behind the eyelids, where they can cause severe pain by pressing on the sensitive cornea (a).

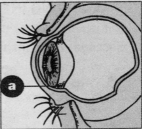

• High-speed metallic foreign bodies can sometimes pass through coats of the eye and lodge in the inside.

◆ **If the body is not easily located,** it may be

helpful to fold the upper lid up over a matchstick to see it (**b**). This is easier if the victim looks steadily downward.

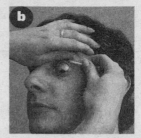

METHODS OF REMOVING
FOREIGN BODIES FROM THE EYE

1 Blinking the eye under water (**a**) or in a full eyebath will often remove a foreign body. **2** A piece of grit on the inside of a lid or near the edge of the cornea can often be picked off with the corner of a folded piece of paper (**b**).

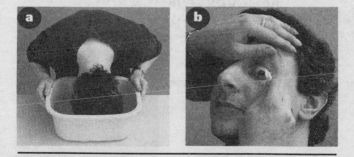

◆ **If the foreign body remains,** then consult a doctor.

✣ **Never use a needle** or other hard pointed object.

✤ **Do not persist** if the grit seems embedded.

✤ **Never try to remove a foreign body** in the center of the cornea. Scarring here will seriously affect vision.

HIGH-SPEED METALLIC FOREIGN BODIES

These tend to come from grindstones, drills, lathes or milling machines and can penetrate the eye almost painlessly, but their presence in the eye is a serious threat to vision. These are a major risk and must be dealt with by an opthalmologist.

FOREIGN BODIES IN THE NOSE

REMOVING FOREIGN BODIES FROM THE NOSE

Small foreign bodies just inside the nostril can often be clearly seen and may sometimes be expelled by blowing the nostril on the affected side. The removal of an obstacle should only be undertaken with extreme caution, and wherever possible, under medical supervision.

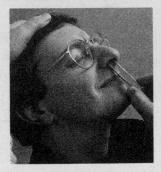

◆ **If the foreign body will still not dislodge,** take the victim to a doctor.

✤ **Do not persist** if not immediately successful, as there is a major risk of pushing the body farther in.

SPLINTERS

REMOVING PROTRUDING SPLINTERS

1 Wood and other splinters should be pulled out with tweezers if a protruding part can be grasped. **2** Wash the area thoroughly with soap and water.

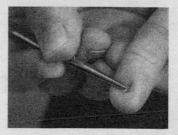

The most common foreign bodies are metal or wood splinters which have become lodged in or under the skin.

SMALL BURIED SPLINTERS

If the splinter is small and buried then use the following method.

REMOVING SMALL BURIED SPLINTERS

1 Sterilize a needle in a flame (**a**). **2** Try to lift up one end of the splinter with the point of the needle (**b**) and then grasp it with tweezers.

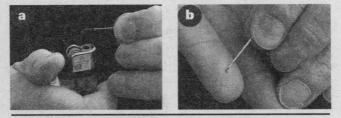

◆ If the splinter will not come out (and especially if the area becomes inflamed), then consult a doctor.

Nausea and vomiting

Nausea and vomiting suggest irritation or distention of the stomach or bowel from any of a number of causes, some of which are listed below. In most cases the vomiting will relieve the symptoms and recovery will occur spontaneously.

CAUSES

• Overeating.

• Excessive alcohol consumption.

• Food poisoning.

• Gastroenteritis.

- Stomach or duodenal ulcer.

- Appendicitis.

RELIEVING NAUSEA AND VOMITING

1 Avoid food. **2** Drink bland liquids only (water or broth), and in small quantities. **3** Note and report other symptoms.

◆ **If the nausea is unexplained** and continues for longer than a day, then call a doctor.

◆ **If the vomiting is unexplained** and continues for more than an hour, then call a doctor.

SUSPECTED POISONING

If there is suspicion of poisoning, a sample of the vomit should be kept for examination.

TRAVEL SICKNESS

Travel sickness is caused by continuous, passive, repetitive body movement in any transport vehicle. It displays the following features.

FEATURES

- Yawning.

- Deep and rapid breathing.

- Salivation.

- Nausea.

- Abdominal discomfort.

- Pallor.

- Sweating.

- Vomiting.

- Headache.

- Dizziness.

- Fatigue.

✤ **Avoid** alcohol consumption and eat only in moderation.

RELIEVING TRAVEL SICKNESS

1 Try to get into the fresh air. **2** Sit down with the head tilted backwards (**a**). **3** If on a boat, fix the eyes on an unmoving point, such as the horizon (**b**).

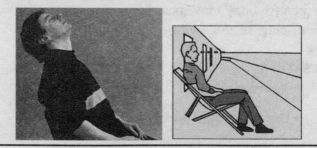

5

Dressings, Bandages and Slings

There are various types of dressings and bandages and a variety of ways in which to apply them, depending on the injury and the materials available. Although dressings and bandages can be bought, it is possible to improvise using towels, handkerchiefs, linen, etc.

♣ **Do not place** fluffy material directly on to a wound, as the fibers will stick to it.

Dressings

A dressing should always be large enough to cover the wound and extend for 2.5 cm (1 in) around it. If possible, it should be sterile so that no bacteria are introduced to the injury. It should also be made of a material that allows the sweat to evaporate. If sweat accumulates, the dressing becomes wet and an ideal environment for bacterial growth is created.

FUNCTIONS

- To protect the wound.

- To control bleeding and to help blood to clot.

- To absorb any fluid from the wound.

- To prevent infection.

APPLYING DRESSINGS: RULES

- The hands should be thoroughly washed.

- The wound and the surrounding skin should be thoroughly cleaned, as long as the wound is not too large and the bleeding has been controlled.

- Use extra cotton wool padding, secured with a bandage, to cover a field dressing. This will absorb excess fluid and help to control bleeding.

- Replace a dressing that may have slipped from the wound to an uncleansed area of skin with a new dressing. This will prevent infection.

- Always place a dressing directly on to a wound.

✤ **Do not slide** a dressing on to a wound from uncleansed skin.

✤ **Do not touch** the wound or any part of the dressing that will come into contact with it.

✤ **Do not talk** or cough over a wound or dressing.

BANDAGES (ADHESIVE DRESSINGS)

These have an adhesive backing (a), to which is attached a square cellulose or gauze pad (b), covered with protective strips (c). It is the pad which is placed directly on to the wound. Bandages are available in sterile wrappings and come in various shapes and sizes. They will not stick to the area around the wound unless it is clean and dry.

A Bandage

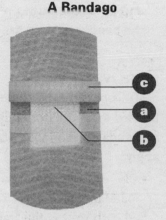

APPLYING A BANDAGE

1 Unwrap the bandage and hold it with the pad downwards. **2** Peel back the two protective strips, but do not remove them (a) and ▶

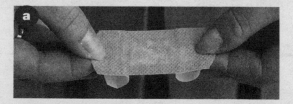

do not touch the gauze pad. **3** Place the gauze pad on the wound. **4** Remove the protective strips completely and press the edges of the bandage down (**b**).

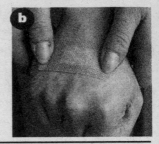

ADHESIVE FABRIC TAPE

Rolls of this tape come in various sizes. It should be used to secure non-adhesive dressings, if there are no bandages available, or if bandages are difficult to apply.

ADHESIVE FABRIC TAPE

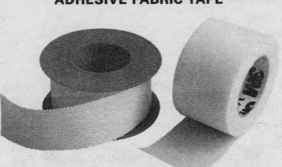

FIELD (STERILE) DRESSINGS

These are dressings which, for the sake of convenience and efficient application, have layers of gauze (**a**) and cotton-wool padding (**b**) already attached to a roller bandage (**c**). These are the best first aid dressings for large wounds. They come in sterile wrappings and are available in various shapes and sizes.

A FIELD DRESSING

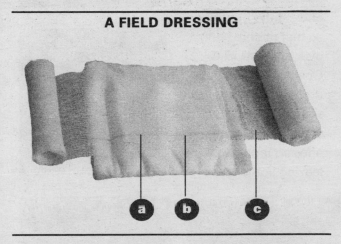

APPLYING A FIELD DRESSING

1 Remove the inner and outer wrappings.
2 The special bandage and folded dressing should be held in one hand. Unravel the short end of the bandage (**a**). **3** Hold the ends of the bandage so that the dressing is over the wound (**b**). Open out the folded dressing. **4** Wrap the short end of the bandage around the affected limb (**c**), leaving some of it ▶

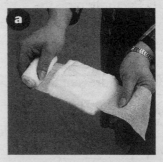

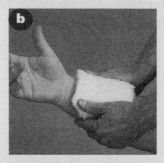

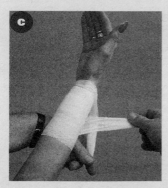

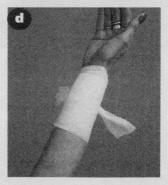

free (to be tied at the end of the procedure).
5 Securely bind the limb with the long end of the bandage until the pad has been covered.
6 Tie the two ends together (**d**) to secure the dressing.

GAUZE DRESSINGS

These are non-adhesive layers of gauze, available in sterile wrappings. They are used for large wounds that need a light covering (e.g., a burn), and can be secured with adhesive tape. If a field dressing is not available, dress the wound in the following way.

GAUZE DRESSINGS

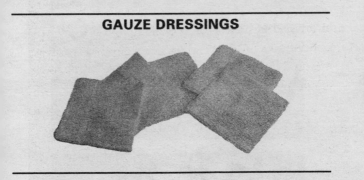

APPLYING A GAUZE DRESSING

1 Unwrap the gauze and hold it by its edges above the wound. **2** Place it on the wound (**a**). **3** Cover the dressing with a pad of cotton wool (**b**). **4** Fix the dressing and cotton wool in place with a roller bandage (**c**) (see pp. 179–182), sticky tape or adhesive fabric tape (see p. 172).

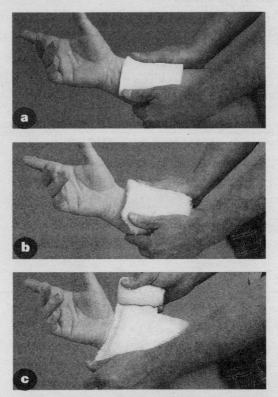

IMPROVISED DRESSINGS

If, in emergency situations, ready-made dressings are not available, any clean, dry, absorbent and non-fluffy material can be used: for example, the inside of a folded handkerchief or a newly washed towel. Folded toilet paper or tissues can also be used. These can then be secured in place with a scarf or some other similar item.

Bandages

Ready-made bandages are generally made from cotton, rayon, elastic net, special paper, etc. There are two main types: roller bandages and triangular bandages.

<u>USES</u>

- To maintain direct pressure and control bleeding.

- To secure dressings.

- To prevent unwanted movement of an injured limb.

- To prevent swelling.

- To support an injured limb or joint.

- To help lift and carry victims.

✤ **Bandages should not** be used for padding if softer materials are available.

APPLYING BANDAGES: RULES

- Apply the bandages while the victim is sitting or lying down.

- Sit or stand in front of the victim and work from his or her injured side.

- Support the injured part in the position in which it is going to be bandaged.

- When the victim is lying down, pass the bandages under the natural hollows of the ankles, knees, back and neck and ease them gently into position.

- If bandages are being used to immobilize a fracture, tie the knots on the uninjured side of the body or limb. If both sides are injured, tie the knots in the center of the affected part.

- If a knot has to be used to secure the bandage, use a reef knot (see p. 197).

- There should be plenty of padding between the limbs and the body, and at bony areas of the limbs (e.g., knees and ankles) before bandaging or immobilizing a fracture.

- The tissues around the injury may swell. Check the bandages frequently to make sure that they are not becoming too tight.

- When bandaging a limb, keep the finger- or toe-nails exposed so that they may be used to check the victim's circulation (see p. 63).

- If using a bandage to maintain direct pressure and to control bleeding, tie a knot over the pad or dressing.

❖ **Bandages should not be so tight** that they interfere with the circulation (see p. 63). They should be firm enough to control bleeding, to keep the dressing in position or to prevent movement.

ROLLER BANDAGES
These are made of cotton, gauze or linen, and are available in rolls of up to 5 m (5 yd). They come in different widths for different parts of the body: finger—2.5 cm (1 in); hand—5 cm (2 in); arm—5 or 6 cm (2 or 2½ in); leg—7.5 or 9 cm (3 or 3½ in); trunk—10 or 15 cm (4 or 6 in). Before the bandages are used, make sure that they are tightly rolled and of a suitable length.

A ROLLER BANDAGE

a head
b tail

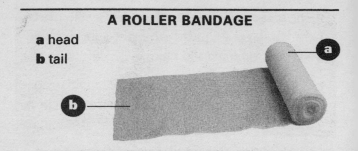

APPLYING ROLLER BANDAGES

SIMPLE SPIRAL BANDAGING

1 Support the injured part by hand in the position in which it is to be bandaged.
2 Hold the bandage with the "head" uppermost. **3** Place the "tail" of the bandage on the limb and begin by bandaging from below the injury upwards and from the inside of the limb outwards. Unroll only a few inches at a time. ▶

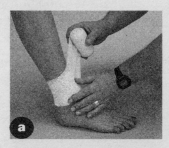

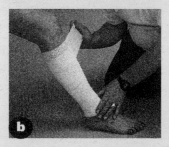

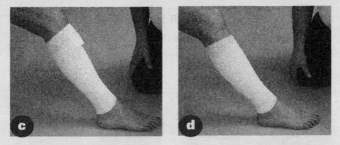

4 Make a firm slanted turn to anchor the bandage (**a**). ▶ **5** Carry on making turns in this way.
Each turn should cover two-thirds of the previous turn, with the edges parallel (**b**). **6** Use a
horizontal turn to begin finishing off. **7** Fold in
the edge of the bandage (**c**). **8** Secure it on the
outside of the limb (or well away from the
injury) (**d**). **9** Check the circulation (see pp. 5
and 63).

✣ If you must apply bandages, do so with care.
Unnecessary movement of the victim may cause
pain and shock. Be particularly careful to avoid
movement at fracture sites.

SECURING A BANDAGE

Bandages may be secured in one of three ways:
• with a safety pin (**a**; see next page);

• with sticky tape or adhesive strapping (**b**; see
  next page);

- by cutting the bandage, wrapping the ends (in opposite directions) around the limb, and tying them together in a reef knot (**c**) (see p. 197).

SECURING A BANDAGE

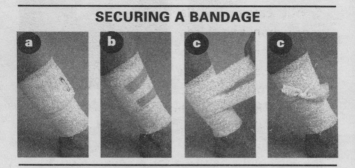

BANDAGING THE KNEE (OR ELBOW)

1 Ask the victim to support the limb in the most comfortable position. **2** Anchor the bandage by holding the tail against one side of the kneecap. **3** Make one straight turn, taking the head over the kneecap and around the joint (**a**). **4** Carry the bandage around the upper leg, covering the top edge of the first turn (**b**). **5** Take the ban- ▶

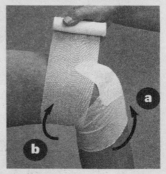

dage around the lower leg covering the lower edge of the first turn. **6** Continue steps 4 and 5 but cover a little more than two thirds of each previous turn. **7** Finish bandaging the joint by using one or

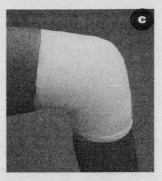

two slanting turns on the upper leg, and securing the bandage on the outside of the leg (**c**). **8** Check the circulation using the toenail test (see p. 63).

BANDAGING THE FOOT AND ANKLE

1 Anchor the bandage by holding its tail underneath the foot, wrapping the bandage around the instep once (**a**). **2** Take the bandage from the top of the instep around the

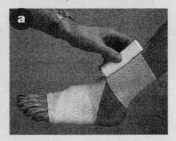

ankle, in a figure-eight pattern, back down over and then underneath the instep (**b**). Overlap each turn so that the instep and heel are covered ▶

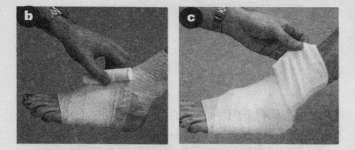

and the ankle supported (**c**). **3** Finish off by using a horizontal turn around the ankle. **4** Secure the folded edge of the bandage on the outside of the ankle.

◆ If it is only the foot that is injured, a turn round the ankle will help to secure the bandage.

BANDAGING THE HAND

1 Ask the victim to support the injured hand with the palm downwards. **2** Anchor the tail of the bandage to the inside of the wrist by making one horizontal turn (**a**). **3** The bandage ▶

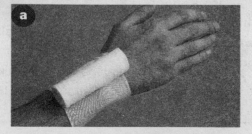

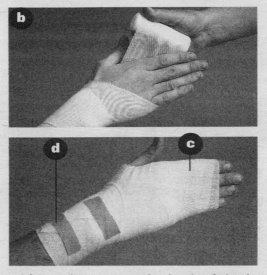

should be taken across the back of the hand
towards the base of the little finger, then
around the palm of the hand under the fingers
(**b**). **4** Take the head of the bandage over the
backs of the fingers horizontally so that its top
edge is aligned with the bottom of the little finger's nail (**c**). **5** Bring the bandage down
around the palm again and diagonally across
the back of the hand towards the wrist.
6 Cover the hand using these figure-eight
turns. **7** Finish with a horizontal turn at the
wrist. **8** Secure the bandage on the back of
the wrist (**d**). **9** Use the fingernail test to check
the circulation (see p. 63).

BANDAGING A SPRAINED WRIST

1 Anchor the tail of the bandage to the wrist with one horizontal turn (**a**).

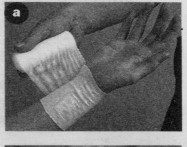

2 Take the bandage diagonally across the palm of the hand, in front of the thumb (**b**).

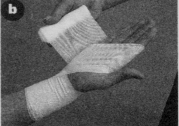

3 Carry the bandage around the back of the hand, across the palm, down to and around the back of the wrist (**c**).

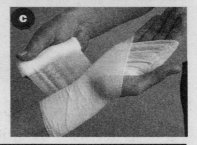

4 Repeat steps 2 and 3 until the wrist is sufficiently supported.

5 Check the circulation (see p. 63).

BANDAGING AROUND FOREIGN BODIES/OPEN FRACTURES

1 Dress the wound (**a**) (see "Open fractures," pp. 125–127).

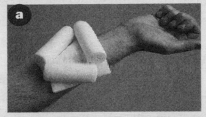

2 Anchor the tail of the bandage under the ring of cotton wool, on the inside of the limb (**b**). **3** Make two horizontal turns to secure the bandage. Bring the head to the top of the cotton wool pad again. **4** Pass

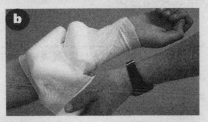

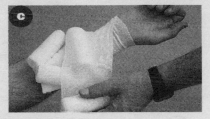

the bandage diagonally under the limb and then up over the pad, avoiding the bone or foreign body (**c**). **5** Take it back down to the start again. **6** Continue steps 4 and 5 until the pad is secure. **7** Check the circulation (see pp. 5 and 63).

WHEN BINDING AN OPEN FRACTURE

Follow steps on p. 187 but make diagonal turns both above and below the ring pad to avoid putting too much pressure on the underside of the fracture.

TRIANGULAR BANDAGES

Although these can be bought, it is possible to make them by cutting a piece of material (such as linen or rayon), of not less than 1 square meter (1 square yard), diagonally in half.

A TRIANGULAR BANDAGE

a point
b end
c base

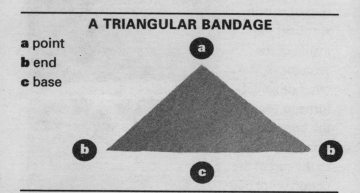

USES

- As slings for support and/or protection.

- For securing dressings on the head, hand or foot.

- To make broad and narrow bandages.

APPLYING TRIANGULAR BANDAGES

BROAD BANDAGES

These are useful for immobilizing fractures.

MAKING BROAD BANDAGES

1 Fold the base, making a narrow hem (**a**).
2 Fold the point towards the base (**b**). **3** Fold the whole bandage in half again in the same direction (**c**).

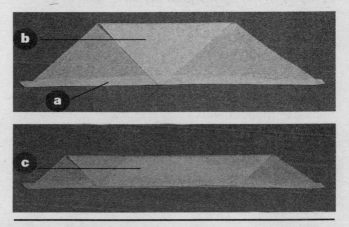

NARROW BANDAGES

These are useful for securing dressings at wrist or ankle joints, if no other type of bandage is available, and for applying as a figure-eight bandage to the feet and ankles when immobilizing a fracture.

MAKING NARROW BANDAGES

1 Make a broad bandage. **2** Fold the broad bandage in half again (towards the base).

APPLYING A FIGURE-EIGHT BANDAGE

1 Pass one end of a narrow bandage under the natural hollows of the ankles, until equal lengths of the bandage lie on either side of the ankles (**a**). **2** Cross the bandage above the ankles (**b**). **3** Wrap the ends around the feet and secure the narrow bandage under the soles of the feet with a reef knot (**c**).

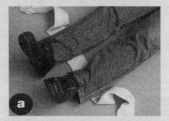

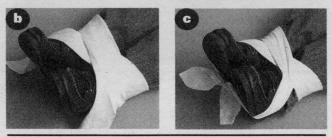

SCALP BANDAGE

Triangular bandages are used on the scalp to hold dressings in place, not to control bleeding.

APPLYING A SCALP BANDAGE

1 Fold a hem along the base of the triangular bandage.

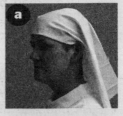

2 Place the bandage so that the center of the base is above the space between the eyebrows (**a**). The point and the ends of the bandage should hang down at the back of the victim's head.

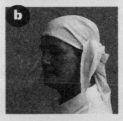

3 Cross the ends of the bandage at back of the head, on top of the point (**b**), and take them round to the front. The point of the triangular bandage should be left hanging down under the crossed-over ends. **4** Tie the ends on the forehead using a reef knot (**c**) (see p. 197). **5** Gently pull the point down, steadying the head with your other hand, to tighten the bandage.

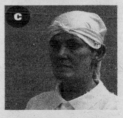

6 Bring the point up and pin it to the bandage on the crown of the head (**d**).

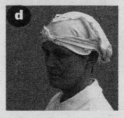

FOOT (OR HAND) BANDAGE

Triangular bandages are used on the hand or foot when dressings need to be held in place, and direct pressure does not need to be maintained.

APPLYING A FOOT (OR HAND) BANDAGE

1 Place the victim's foot on a triangular bandage, so that the point is pointing away from the victim, in the direc-

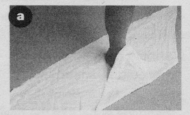

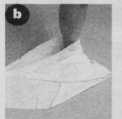
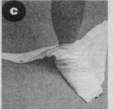
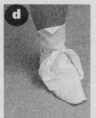

tion of the toes and fingers, and the base (when folded upwards) covers the victim's heel and ankle (or heel of the hand) (**a**). **2** Bring the point up so that it is resting on the lower half of the shin. **3** Bring the ends of the bandage to the front of the foot, cross them over. **4** Take the ends behind the ankle, cross them over, bringing them around to the front again (**b**). **5** Tie them in a reef knot over the ▶

point (**c**). **6** Fold the point over the knot, and secure it to the bandage over the instep with a safety pin (**d**).

Slings

There are two types of sling: the arm sling and the elevation sling. They should always be applied from the injured side, as the first aider is then in a position to support the limb during application.

USES

- To support and protect injured limbs.

- To prevent the movement of an arm when there are chest injuries.

ARM SLING

This type of sling is only effective if the casualty sits or stands. It keeps the forearm in place across the chest. If correctly applied, the victim's hand will be a little higher than the elbow and the fingers, from the lower knuckles onwards, should be visible.

APPLYING AN ARM SLING

1 The casualty should sit down. Ask him or her to support his or her own arm once you have positioned it, with the hand a little ▶

higher than the elbow.
2 Taking one end of a triangular bandage, slide one end between the forearm and chest until the point is level with the elbow but with some material

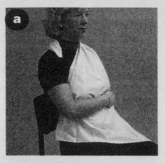

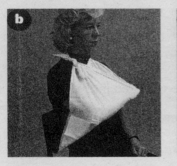
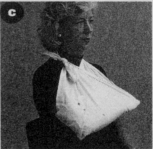

overlapping. **3** Draw the top end up over the shoulder on the uninjured side, round behind the neck, and down over the shoulder on the injured side (**a**). **4** Bring the lower end up over the forearm and secure it to the other end (**b**) with a reef knot (see p. 197) tied just above the collarbone. **5** Bring the point forward and pin it to the front of the bandage (**c**). **6** Check the circulation (see pp. 5 and 63) and adjust the bandage and/or sling if necessary.

♣ **Support the forearm** throughout this procedure.

ELEVATION SLING

This type of sling is used when the hand is bleeding, or if there are shoulder or chest injuries of a complex nature. If applied correctly, the hand should be in a well-raised position.

APPLYING AN ELEVATION SLING

1 Follow step 1 (p. 193) for applying an ordinary arm sling. **2** Position an open triangular bandage over the forearm so that one end covers the hand, several inches of which reach beyond the finger tips. The point should cover the elbow with plenty of overlap (**a**). **3** Gently put the base of the bandage under the ▶

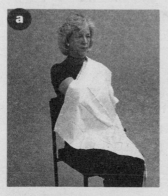
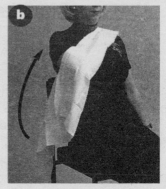

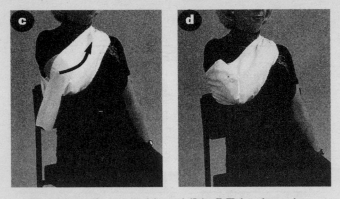

forearm, elbow and hand (**b**). **4** Take the other end around the victim's back and over the shoulder on the uninjured side. Hold the end in place. **5** With your other hand, very gently draw up the end over the fingers of the injured limb to meet the end lying over the shoulder (**c**). **6** Tie the ends together in a reef knot (see p. 197) just above the collarbone. **7** Tuck the point between the arm and the front of the sling. **8** Pin the fold to the sling over the upper arm (**d**).

REF KNOTS

TYING REEF KNOTS

1 Hold one end of the bandage in each hand. **2** Take the left end over and then under the right end (**a**). **3** Take what is now the right end over and under the left end (**b**). **4** Pull the knot tight (**c**).

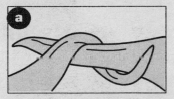

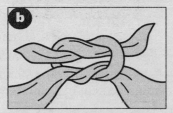

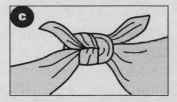

6

Useful Aids

First Aid Kit

Kits can be bought from a drugstore. One can easily be made, however. The contents of a first aid kit should be kept in a suitable plastic container, such as a large sandwich box with a good, tight-fitting and secure lid. This makes the kit suitable both for traveling and for being kept in the medicine cabinet at home. A list of items that you may wish to include is given below.

- 2 large, 2 small sealed, sterile field dressings for covering wounds.
- 1 large packet of sterile, sealed bandages (adhesive dressings) of large size.
- 1 packet of smaller sterile, sealed bandages (adhesive dressings) of various sizes.
- 2 sealed packets of 10 sterile 10 cm x 10 cm (4 in x 4 in) plain gauze for dressing wounds.
- 1 roll of 2.5 cm (1 in) wide elastoplast or rayon adhesive tape.

- 1 flat tin of sterile paraffin-coated gauze for blisters and large grazes.
- 3 triangular bandages for immobilizing fractures and sprains.
- 4 large, open-weave gauze bandages.
- 2 packets of sterile cotton wool swabs for cleaning cuts, grazes, etc.
- 2 rolls of non-sterile cotton wool, for cleaning wounds and for padding.
- 1 bottle of acetaminophen pain reliever tablets.
- 1 clinical thermometer.
- 1 pair of flat-ended tweezers, without serrations, for removing foreign bodies.
- 1 pair of scissors, with round ends for cutting bandages and gauze.
- Safety pins of various sizes.
- 1 plastic bottle of antiseptic solution for cleaning wounds, cuts and grazes.
- 1 tube of hydrocortisone cream for insect bites, hives, etc.
- *HarperEssentials First Aid.*

Medicines in the Home

Prescription and non-prescription medicines should be kept in a safe place. A cupboard that is in a cool, dry place, well out of reach of children and fitted with a child-proof lock makes the ideal medicine cabinet. Only medical aids should be kept inside it. Medicines should always be stored in the medicine cabinet and never left lying around. They should be safely disposed of if they have expired or no longer used.

CONTENTS OF THE MEDICINE CABINET

- Emergency telephone numbers: doctor, hospital and local drugstore.

- First aid kit.

- Prescription and non-prescription medicines.

COMMON PROBLEMS AND MEDICINAL REMEDIES

Problem	Remedy
Bites and stings	Hydrocortisone cream
Colds	Decongestant nose drops or tablets Antihistamine tablets
Cuts and grazes	Antiseptic cream or solution
Constipation	Laxatives: osmotics (e.g., Ex-lax); lubricants (e.g., glycerine suppositories)
Diarrhea	Anti-diarrheal drugs (e.g., Kaopectate)
Fever	Temperature-lowering drugs: aspirin; acetaminophen (adult and children's strength)
Sore throat	Throat lozenges and antiseptic mouthwash
Sunburn and rash	Anti-inflammatory lotions and creams: calamine lotion; hydrocortisone cream
Wound cleaning	Antiseptic solution

GUIDE TO ADMINISTERING MEDICINES

Non-prescription medicines. With medicines that are sold over the counter, the directions for taking them should be read very carefully.

Prescription medicines. With these, find out from your doctor or pharmacist whether

- they can be used with alcohol;

- they induce sleep;

- it is safe to drive or operate machinery while taking them;

- they can be used with the contraceptive pill;

- there are any other medicines or foods that should not be taken at the same time.

Also, check

- when and how often they should be taken;

- whether or not they can be taken on an empty stomach, and how long after a meal a person should wait before taking them.

DRUGS GLOSSARY

Analgesics Pain relieving drugs, such as aspirin, acetaminophen and ibuprofen.

❖ **Children under 12** should not be given aspirin except on medical advice.

Antibiotics These are drugs that can kill bacteria. They can be taken internally or applied to the skin.

  ✤ Overuse of **antibiotics** can mean a risk of an allergic reaction or the development of antibiotic-resistant bacteria.

Anti-convulsants These control epilepsy.

Anti-depressants These drugs are mood altering, and are prescribed to depressed people.

Anti-diabetic drugs These stimulate the production of insulin or are taken to replace it.

Anti-diarrheal drugs These are used to manage diarrhea. They slow the action of the bowel or make the stools more solid.

Anti-emetics These are used to treat nausea and vomiting.

Antihistamines These reduce swelling, and are used internally to treat allergies, asthma, insect bites and stings, and hives. They are also used to prevent travel sickness.

  ✤ **Antihistamines can cause** drowsiness and this may be dangerously increased if alcohol is taken.

Antispasmodics These stop muscles from going into spasms. They relax the muscles of the intestines and lungs, and are used to treat some types of asthma.

Barbiturates These are sedatives which depress brain activity.

❖ **Barbiturates are habit forming** and widely abused.

Benzodiazepines See Tranquilizers (below).

Corticosteroids These are used to reduce inflammation externally and internally. They are available as nose drops, sprays (for asthma), hydrocortisone creams, injections and oral preparations.

❖ **Large amounts** taken internally can mean loss of calcium from the bones, an increase in weight, abnormal skin markings and a roundness in the shape of the face.

Diuretics These drugs encourage urination.

Heart and blood pressure drugs Digitalis drugs are used to treat heart failure, and irregular and rapid heartbeat. Blood pressure drugs include diuretics.

Laxatives These drugs encourage the passing of stools. They act in three ways: by increasing the bulk of the stools; by softening and lubricating the stools; by stimulating bowel action.

Tranquilizers These are used to treat anxiety, together with anti-depressants. They include the benzodiazepines (e.g., Valium).

❖ **Tranquilizers are physically** addictive if taken for more than a month.

❖ **Alcohol should not** be drunk when using these drugs.